A COMPREHENSI

To lose weight, boo
detoxify your

70+ Delicious Recipes & Bonus :
21-Day Meal Plan + 6 weeks Planner

INTERMITTENT
FASTING
FOR WOMEN OVER 50

DIANE GAIN

TABLE OF CONTENTS

INTRODUCTION

50 years is a delicate moment in a woman's life. We feel complete, we have accumulated experiences and emotions. We've got involved countless times, made mistakes, and learned from them. And when we felt like we had found certain stability and balance, things started to change again. Menopause is approaching and is questioning our certainties and our balances. But we have learned that changes are not always to be feared, because they can bring with them pleasant surprises and new awareness. My goal with this book is precisely to help the women who are preparing to face this phase, of life, giving them theoretical and practical tools. Menopause, like every other stage of our life, is not difficult, but it could become difficult if we do not have the right tools. I would like you to be aware that our strength, our potential, and our beauty will always accompany us.

Our body is about to enter a new phase where hormones start working in different ways. For this reason, we may feel a little disoriented, having never experienced these sensations before. It starts to change the way we deal with certain situations.

It cannot be denied that with the passage of time some processes in our organism begin to mutate: metabolism slows down and we may experience weight gain; some parts of the body begin to deteriorate giving rise to inflammatory processes or localized pain; we may notice the difference in how our digestive system assimilates foods and experience a lower level of energy. You might find that things you could eat with no issue as recently as five years ago, are suddenly giving you heartburn or they can cause unwanted effects. For many of these, it strikes us as a cruel aspect of reality and it seems like we're moving past the things that we enjoy in life and that we're relegated to less interesting meals. But precisely because I believe that food is one of the pleasures of life, I have inserted at the end of the book an entire chapter dedicated to tasty and simple recipes that will allow you to enjoy your meals with joy and at the same time take care of your well-being. Maybe this will require a small change of perspective from you but I am sure it will be worth it.

While this is a negative frame of mind, I completely understand it and you're entitled to feel that way at first. It is important to know, however, that your metabolism and your body are simply shifting into a different phase and that you've got a lot of other things going on, especially hormone-wise. You will find that things like menopause and certain other aspects of the aging process are the reasons we have to adjust a lot of things. You might be surprised to learn that the things you eat do have a bearing on how you're feeling and they do have a bearing on how quickly and easily your body adapts to those changes. I'm not saying they're solely responsible, simply that the fuel you're giving your body does make a difference.

In this context, intermittent fasting proves to be a very powerful tool. Through this practice, in fact, for reasons that I will exhaustively explain in the next chapters, it is possible to balance the entire metabolism, solve some dysfunctions and surprisingly increase the level of energy.

With intermittent fasting, your focus is not only on the structure you use for your meal consumption but also on ensuring that your body is getting all of the required nutrients it needs in order to function properly while you're eating. If you commit to doing the intermittent fasting regime, you must also commit to making sure that your meals contain all the correct ingredients to sustain you, to activate the right hormone production in your body, and the supplemental nutrition you will need to make the very best of the time your body is spending breaking down the fat stores in your body for crucial nutrition and energy.

While your body is making these adjustments in the way it's continuing to regenerate cells for hair, skin, organs, etc., it is making use of the food you're giving it in order to do those things. If you're able to provide your body with the ideal balance of macro-nutrients (fat, protein, and carbohydrates) from ideal and nourishing sources, you will find that your body simply thrives on what it's been given. You will find that the processes in your body—everything from the simple stuff like sleeping to the more complex stuff like organ health—will continue on with more ease.

Some women in this age group have found themselves grappling with things that were never a problem for them before. Some women find that in spite of the fact that they were carrying on through their days while feeling like they could fall asleep standing up at any moment, they are completely unable to sleep when the time finally comes for them to hang up their hats for the day. Some women find that around the time they would typically be menstruating, their bodies are throwing curveballs at them that are simply impossible to anticipate. Some women find that their digestive system simply won't process things in the way that it once did.

Our bodies at this point of our lives, tend to require a much higher balance of elements such as vitamins, minerals, fiber, and things that tend to be forgotten in the everyday diet unless you've spent a lot of time being very health-conscious. Many of us have simply been busy living our lives, minding what we eat, exercising when we can, without breaking down the daily values and percentages of everything we eat to find out what works best. Most of us haven't planned our diets using any scientific method, figuring out what measures of certain nutrients are better than others.

While intermittent fasting doesn't go that far, it can certainly feel like that in the beginning, and it is crucial that you be on the lookout for the changes in your body and your overall wellness to ensure that you're making changes for the better and that your body is gaining benefits from the methods and foods you're using on a daily basis.

For women our age, it can seem like there are just a lot of things going on in our bodies all at once and you really wouldn't be wrong in assuming that. Where you might be mistaken in your assumption, however, is that it doesn't need to be the end of the world and it doesn't have to be very hard to turn the ship around. You have many years ahead of you and you have a lot left to do here with life, family, goals, and all the things you have worked so hard for in your life.

Life is meant to be enjoyed and that does not change, no matter what age you've reached. Intermittent fasting is here to give you the tools to make life enjoyable so you can continue to do what makes life worth living without having to suffer at the hands of changing bodily processes and hormone outputs!

WHY DOES IT HELP?

I will guide you step by step towards understanding the changes taking place within our body at this stage of life, and I will make available to you all the information necessary to build a personalized path of healing and slimming according to your personal needs.

Choosing to fast at intermittent periods throughout your week can give you an advantage that allows your metabolism to change for the better, allows you to cut down your intake throughout the week, and can help you feel your best. Throughout history and cultures all across the globe, you will see references to and instances of fasting. This is influenced by a number of factors throughout history, but the main one is the scarcity of food.

It just so happens that our bodies are accustomed to the periodic scarcity of food and can thrive on it more than we may previously have believed. When we give our body intermittent periods of food scarcity, our bodies are forced to sustain themselves retrieving from the fat storages that our bodies have accumulated over the years.

Excess glucose that is taken on by the body is stored as fat to be used later. This is the mechanism that allowed humankind to survive those periodic stages of food scarcity and our bodies are still operating in that same way. You might notice that your body has some stores of fat that it keeps around a little longer than you might like. That's because your body is waiting for its perfect opportunity to put those reserves to use! By doing intermittent fasting, you give your body every opportunity to put those reserves to use and to subsist off of them, without depriving your body of the essential nutrients it needs in order to thrive and survive.

By making sure that the meals you eat are healthy, wholesome, and packed with all the right nutrients, you're making sure that your body isn't simply starving during the times when you're not eating. It's got plenty of energy to use with the stores of fat in your body, and it's got all the nutrients from the supplements and the whole foods you're eating.

The hormonal changes in your body are what allow you to get access to those stores of fat and break them down for energy. In addition to this, you will find that your sensitivity to insulin will improve. If you have difficulties with your insulin tolerance or the stability of your blood sugar levels, you might find that doing intermittent fasting is helpful for this.

Many people who have trouble with their blood sugar regularity will find they have trouble with keeping themselves from crashing in the early afternoon. People who struggle with that might find that they have trouble staying full until their next meal and may even feel a little bit of light-headedness or mood swings between meals. This could be the indication of something a little more serious depending on how difficult it is for you to sustain yourself between mealtimes, so be sure that your doctor is checking your A1C for evidence of diabetes.

If you have found that you do have type II diabetes that developed as a result of certain eating habits, it is something that can typically be reversed with the help of a structured diet that contains more of the foods your body needs in order to survive and less of the foods that interfere with your body's use of insulin. In such cases, however, you will want to ensure that you are taking on the right foods in the right quantities to support you between meals, meaning you might need to start your fasting on a much more stringent and abbreviated timeline with the help of your doctor.

Many people who are working to turn around their diabetes have found that, with a specially-planned regimen, they were able to work toward an intermittent fasting schedule while they worked to improve their diabetes or insulin sensitivity. By filling your body with 2,000 or fewer calories of whole, nutritious, low-glycemic foods, you might find that your condition will improve and your ability to stabilize your blood sugar for several hours at a time will improve along with that, allowing you to branch out to and get onto an intermittent fasting regimen that works for you!

CHAPTER 1

WHAT IS INTERMITTENT FASTING?

Basically, Fasting is defined as abstaining from eating anything. It is the deliberate action of depriving the body of any form of food for more than six hours.

Whereas Intermittent fasting is a nutritional strategy that provides for a more or less long interval of fasting over a few days, alternating with a period in which you can take food without being too enslaved to the weights but still taking into account some precautions. Intermittent fasting does not need to be carried out every day, but you can choose the different ways suitable for your goals and lifestyles.

In the hours of feeding it is possible to consume almost all foods giving preference to low-calorie foods such as meat, fish, eggs, limiting simple sugars and choosing those with a low glycemic index, bread pasta, and rice possibly whole grains, legumes, dried and fresh fruits, good fats

One of its forms where the fast is carried out in a cyclic manner with the aim to reduce the overall caloric intake in a day.

The main goal is to divert the body's attention from the digestion of food. During the fasting period, in fact, a series of metabolic changes take place in the body: since there is no food left in the stomach to digest, the body focuses on the process of recovery and maintenance.

To most people, it may sound unhealthy and damaging for the body, but scientific research has proven that fasting can produce positive results on the human mind and body. According to Healthline, the American medical-scientific journal, this system helps reduce overall calorie intake and as a result not only can help people lose weight effortlessly but can improve the overall functioning of metabolism. It can also positively affect our mind teaching self-discipline and fights against bad eating practices and habits. It is basically an umbrella term that is used to define all voluntary forms of fasting. This dietary approach does not restrict the consumption of certain food items; rather, it works by reducing the overall food intake, leaving enough space to meet the essential nutrients the body needs. Therefore, it is proven to be far more effective and much easier in implementation, given that the dieter completely understands the nature and science of intermittent fasting.

Intermittent fasting is categorized into three broad methods of food abstinence, including alternate-day fasting, daily restrictions, and periodic fasting. The means may vary, but the end goal of intermittent fasting remains the same, which is to achieve a better metabolism, healthy body weight, and active lifestyle. The American Heart Association, AHA, has also studied intermittent fasting and its results. According to the AHA, it can help in countering insulin resistance, cardio-metabolic diseases, and leads to weight loss. However, a question mark remains on the sustainability of this health-effective method. The 2019 research "Effects of intermittent fasting on health, aging, and disease" has also found intermittent fasting to be effective against insulin resistance, inflammation, hypertension, obesity, and dyslipidemia. However, the work on this dietary approach is still underway, and the traditional methods of fasting which existed for almost the entire human history, in every religion from Buddhism to Jainism, Orthodox

Christianity, Hinduism, and Islam, are studied to found relevance in today's age of science and technology.

How Does It Work

Eating is a primary need that we satisfy unceasingly from birth. Every day we introduce food into our organism. When we eat, the metabolism activates itself to start the digestive process. This process uses a huge amount of energy. The more food we introduce, the more the body will have to work to metabolize it. If the food is introduced and too much, or too full of sugars and fats the effort that the digestive system must sustain and yet greater.

When we fast, however, we stop this process and this energy dispendium. The saved energy is thus diverted to other metabolic processes, essentially of a restorative type.

Dr. Longo, Director of the Institute of Longevity at the University of Southern California, explained how, thanks to this practice: "the immune system frees itself from useless, unnecessary cells, while it is driven to put back into action naturally, as was the case at the moments of birth and growth, stem cells capable of ensuring regeneration".

The body not engaged in food digestion can better devote itself to its purification by moving toxins away through its emunctory organs. These large internal cleanings obviously have positive repercussions on the state of health of organs and tissues. The organism is detoxified and revitalized.

American researchers at Yale's School of Medicine highlighted how during the break from food, our organism produces a substance capable of extinguishing chronic inflammation. It is called the β-hydroxybutyrate (BHB) and it is capable turn falls into a complex set of proteins that guide the inflammatory response in many pathologies, including several autoimmune diseases. A good result suggests how in the future therapeutic fasting can be used in the early treatment of many inflammatory-based diseases.

Intermittent fasting is a tool that can help us activate the processes described above and face a real fast. In fact, it works between alternating periods of eating and fasting. It is a much more flexible approach, as there are many options to choose from according to body type, size, weight goals, and nutritional needs.

The human body works like a synchronized machine that requires sufficient time for self-healing and repair. When we constantly eat junk and unhealthy food or too high a quantity of food without the consideration of our caloric needs, it leads to obesity and toxic build-up in the body. That is why fasting comes as a natural means of detoxifying the body and providing it enough time to utilize its fat deposits.

Whatever the human body consumes is ultimately broken into glucose, which is later utilized by the cells in glycolysis to release energy. As the blood glucose level rises, insulin is produced to lower the levels and allow the liver to carry out De Novo Lipogenesis, the process in which the excess glucose is turned into glycogen and ultimately stored into fat, resulting in obesity. Intermittent fasting seems to reverse this process by deliberately creating energy deprivation, which is then fulfilled by breaking down the existing fat deposits.

Intermittent fasting works through lipolysis; though it is a natural body process, it can only be initiated when the blood glucose levels drop to a sufficiently low point. That point can be achieved through fasting and exercising. When a person cuts off the external glucose supply for several hours, the body switches to lipolysis. This process of breaking the fats also releases other by-products like ketones which are capable of reducing the oxidative stress of the body and help in its detoxification.

Mark Mattson, a neuroscientist from the Johns Hopkins Medicine University, has studied intermittent fasting for almost 25 years of his career. He laid out the workings of intermittent fasting by clarifying its clinical application and the science behind it. According to him, intermittent fasting must be opted for a healthy lifestyle.

While discussing the application of this dietary approach, it is imperative to understand how intermittent fasting stands out from casual dieting practices. It is not mere abstinence from eating. What is eaten in this dietary lifestyle is equally important as the fasting itself. It does not result in malnutrition; rather, it promotes healthy eating along with the fast. Intermittent fasting is divided into two different states that follow one another. The cycle starts with the "FED" state, which is followed by a "Fasting" state. The duration of the fasting state and the frequency of the FED state are established by the method of intermittent fasting. The latter is characterized by high blood glucose levels, whereas during the fasting state the body goes through a gradual decline in glucose levels. This decline in glucose signals the pancreas and the brain to meet the body's energy needs by processing the available fat molecules. However, if the fasting state is followed by a FED state in which a person binge eats food rich in carbs and fats, it will turn out to be more hazardous for their health. Therefore, the fasting period must be accompanied by a healthy diet.

THE SCIENCE BEHIND INTERMITTENT FASTING

Biologically, intermittent fasting works at many levels, from cellular levels to gene expression and body growth. In order to understand the science behind the workings of intermittent fasting, it is important to learn about the role of insulin levels, human growth hormones, cellular repair, and gene expression.

Intermittent fasting firstly lowers glucose levels, which in turn drops insulin levels. This lowering of insulin helps fat burning in the body, thus gradually curbing obesity and related disorders. Controlled levels of insulin are also responsible for preventing diabetes and insulin resistance. On the other hand, intermittent fasting boosts the production of human growth hormones up to five times. The increased production of HGH aids quick fat burning and muscle formation.

During the fasting state, the body goes into the process of self-healing at cellular levels, thus removing the unwanted, unfunctional cells and debris. This creates a cleansing effect that directly or indirectly nourishes the body and allows it to grow under reduced oxidative stress. Likewise, fasting even affects the gene expression within the human body. The cell functions according to the coding and decoding of the gene's expression; when this transcription occurs at a normal pace in a healthy environment, it automatically translates into the longevity of the cells, and fasting ensures unhindered transcription. Thus, intermittent fasting fights aging, cancer, and boosts the immune system by strengthening the body cells.

HISTORY OF INTERMITTENT FASTING

Often confused with starvation, fasting is not a recent concept; it is as old as the known human history. It is completely natural and much needed for body development. Even the word "breakfast" itself indicates that we normally fast between two meals of the day. Intermittent fasting takes this process to the next step and sets up a dietary routine that works best for bodily health.

Fasting, in one form or another, remained widely prevalent in every ancient civilization because of its obvious benefits. We often hear stories of monks acquiring spiritual superiority and physical strength through fasts. The tradition existed even from 460 to 370 BC, the times of Hippocrates, which is today considered the pioneer of modern medicine. He prescribed two basic methods to achieve physical healing: one was fasting, and the other was the intake of apple cider vinegar.

"To eat when you are sick is to feed your illness" – (Hippocrates of Kos)

Those words of Hippocrates laid the basis of intermittent fasting, which is equally relevant today. His ideas about fasting and its benefits were also shared by other Greek physicians and writers of the time like Plutarch, who, between 46-120 AD, preached the concept of fasting by describing it as a better approach to treat illness than the use of medicines. Likewise, other great names of Greece, Aristotle, and Plato also supported the concept of fasting and implemented it during their lifetimes.

According to the ancient Greek experts, fasting can be described as the 'physician within' oneself because when a person falls ill, the body naturally loses the appetite to eat, which means that healing can be carried out when a person is fasting. Feeling anorexic when you are sick is natural, and only supports the need for fasting. Thus, with the historical evidence alongside a biological understanding of the human body, it can be inferred that fasting is an essential requirement of every individual and helps in improving health. Besides physical fitness, fasting was also considered an effective means of boosting the cognitive potential of a person, according to Greek physicists. When a person is on the fast, the body and mind go into an ultra-alter mode as most of the blood is supplied to the brain instead of the digestive system. This is the reason why a person feels drowsy and lethargic when he consumes a large amount of food at a time because all the energy and the blood are supplied to digest the food.

Another great supporter of fasting is the founder of toxicology - Philip Paracelsus, who followed in the footsteps of Hippocrates and Galen by writing excessively about the benefits of fasting. He also termed it the physician within - the greatest remedy. Moving forward to the modern medicinal history of America, from 1706 -1790, Benjamin Franklin also highlighted fasting and resting as two better approaches than medicine.

Fasting is also supported by almost all the major religions in the world. Therefore, we find that the respective followers in each religious cult are keeping fasts. According to different religions like Christianity, Jainism, Hinduism, Buddhism, and Islam, fasting is directly linked to spiritual upliftment. It is also described as a means of getting control of the body and its desires. This is where religion and science meet when it comes to fasting, a better control of the body means a person can make wise and healthy food choices for oneself.

Though fasting has always been in use, the contemporary approach of intermittent fasting emerged in 2012, when it was readily picked up by health experts all around the world, and is now widely recommended to people suffering from different health issues. It all started with one single documentary "Eat Fast, Live longer and Book the Fast diet," presented by Dr. Michael Mosley. He was followed by Kate Harrison who wrote a complete book on one of the fasting methods, named the 5:2 diet. Soon in 2016, Dr. Jason Fung stepped up with his book The Obesity Code, which was also marked as the bestseller of that year. In his book, Fung extensively wrote about his own experience with intermittent fasting and how it can be most effective by pairing it with a suitable healthy diet. He recommended the use of fresh vegetables, fruits, protein-rich food, low-carb items, and intake of healthy fats in the diet.

Steadily, all this work on intermittent fasting made enough buzz that people, in general, started opting for its various approaches. Initially, it was just television or movie celebrities who followed the fasting patterns. Then they became the source of inspiration for millions of others.

BENEFITS OF INTERMITTENT FASTING

- CELLULAR REPAIR
- REDUCE INFLAMMATION
- INTESTINAL MICROBIOTA RENEWAL
- LOWERS INSULIN
- LOWERS BLOOD PRESSURE
- IMPROVE HEARTH HEALTH

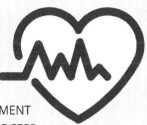

- IMMUNE SYSTEM IMPROVEMENT
- ACTIVATE SELF HEALING PROCESS
- IMPROVE FUNCTIONALITY OF ALL ORGANS
- ALLEVIATE OSSIDATIVE STRESS

- SUSTAINABLE FAT LOSS
- ANTI AGING PROCESS
- BETTER SLEEP
- BETTER MOOD

SELF-HEALING

Intermittent fasting is a great tool for your body to activate your "self-healing" operations. When you are continuously eating, you are not giving your body and your cells the time they need to rest. They need this time to repair themselves or dispose of those cells that may get tainted or destructive. This procedure is called autophagy and can be triggered under specific intermittent fasting conditions.

As Hippocrates has already argued, the human organism has extraordinary capabilities and possesses the innate ability to regenerate and self-regulate. Healing is a spontaneous process that the organism implements autonomously if put in a position to do so. The natural state of balance of every living being and health and not a disease. According to the principles of Hippocratic medicine, we should conceive healing as a process through realigning our body and mind to the laws of Mother Nature.

Through intermittent fasting, it is possible to support the organism in implementing such a function naturally. This is certainly the main mechanism triggered by the fasting that starts all other re-praved processes as a chain reaction.

DEFECTIVE CELL CLEANING

Intermittent fasting promotes autophagy, which is how the body disposes of cells that are more likely to get contaminated or become destructive. Faulty cells not performing at the highest level can accelerate aging, as well as Alzheimer's disease, and type 2 diabetes.

The repairing procedure can be increased during intermittent fasting as the body does not need to concentrate on food assimilation. It can instead, completely focus on cell repair. This procedure is called autophagy.

During fasting, by ceasing digestion all energy of the organism is used for the disposal of toxins, stimulating a significant increase in the cleansing process with healing power.

By fasting, the body can't take energy from food but has to take it elsewhere. And so it is forced to find another survival technique. Its strategy is to turn to reserves: inspect all tissues to recover fats, proteins, vitamins, and minerals that we have available in our internal storage.

Being forced to rummage through the reserves, it analyzes all the textures in search of useful nutrients. When it performs this action, if it finds damaged or excess tissues it eliminates them. This process is called autolysis. The damaged tissues are then replaced by new tissues created by the organism itself. All non-recyclable elements, such as toxins that have no use for survival, are simply eliminated. So we can state that the fasting action is dedicated to renewal.

ACTIVATING CELLULAR REPAIR

Fasting has been known to kick-start the body's natural cellular repair function, get rid of mature cells, increase longevity, and improve hormone function. All things that tend to become problems as people age. This can alleviate joint and muscle aches as well as lower back pain. As the cells are being repaired and the damage is undone, it helps with the skin's elasticity and health.

DIGESTIVE SYSTEM REPAIR

During fasting, the digestive canal does not work, and the digestive mucous membranes can repair themselves. The stomach rebuilds its walls, the glands purify. The liver eliminates fat, in addition to the calculations and slag that congest it. Fasting also allows the regeneration of the intestine by eliminating the slag that hindered it. In this way, its bacterial flora returns to equilibrium. The occlusions disappear. Cleaning the intestinal membrane generates better assimilation of food to the blood.

This process is very important because it can often happen that even if we eat foods rich in vitamins, amino acids, mineral salts, etc. correctly and in the right amount, our body, which is too intoxicated, has difficulty absorbing and using them in the best way. Fasting cleans the intestines and therefore also improves the absorption of the resources it has at its disposal.

I would like to remind you that filling the stomach does not mean feeding. I can eat large quantities of food without receiving nutrients. This happens for example if I eat a portion of French fries, more pasta, more pizza. I am introducing a lot of food, I feel satiated but in fact, I meet malnutrition, since not all the components useful for a state of well-being of the body have been introduced in a balanced way such as: vitamins of various groups, good fats, noble proteins, antioxidants.

I feel obligated to point out that despite intermittent fasting providing you with very important benefits (which I will explain in detail in the next pages), it is also important to know the basic rules of a healthy diet, in order to apply them in the respective time frame when (depending on the respective fasting protocol that you choose) it is allowed to eat. For this reason, in the last chapter of this book, you will find a wide range of recipes as an additional tool to your intermittent fasting pathway.

Some scientific studies report that people examined during the fasting period have achieved important changes of all metabolic parameters such as blood sugar, cholesterol, triglycerides, and insulin, without changing their eating habits, only by fasting. However, I firmly believe that if we support our intermittent fasting protocol with a more natural type of diet, rich in fresh and non-industrial foods, with a strong limitation of sugary drinks and refined flours, we make our detox process much more effective and beneficial both for the body and for the mind.

IMMUNE SYSTEM IMPROVEMENT

By finding new energy, thanks to fasting, the intestine dedicates itself to its cleaning. In this way, it eliminates all slag, outbreaks, and microbes. This translates into greater efficiency of our immune system. This is because fasting forces the body to use sugar and fat reserves and destroy a significant portion of white blood cells. This elimination of white blood cells causes the body to produce new cells within our immune system. Using the words of Dr. Valter Longo, abstinence from food ignites a kind of 'regenerative switch' that pushes stem cells to create new white blood cells, thus regenerating the entire immune system.

As many of you may know, the intestine is considered our second brain, precisely because the well-being not only of our immune system, but also of our mind, depends on its state. We must never forget that in the holistic vision body and mind are a single entity. So the health of the former is reflected in the well-being of the second.

BLOOD PRESSURE

Blood pressure indicates the measure of the strength that blood exerts on the arteries as it flows through our veins. Usually the pressure increases and decreases during the day. But if it remains constantly elevated it can damage the heart causing: heart disease, cognitive decline and dementia, kidney disease, decreased vision, and heart attack. Using the 130/80 measurement, the AHA estimates that 103 million American adults suffer from high blood pressure.

By fasting, our body destroys and eliminates slag, including cholesterol deposits, fat plaques in the arteries, stones, and dead cells. All this has a huge benefit on the blood. We are seeing a considerable decrease in triglycerides and cholesterol. This involves the release of blood vessels, therefore of greater blood flow, the consequent regularization of blood pressure, so those suffering from hypertension can definitely benefit from fasting.

In the early 2000s, a study on the benefits of fasting showed that this not only reduced blood pressure in a group of 174 study participants, but that the effects were lasting. Participants who had pressure values above 140/90 were subjected to a water-only fast under medical supervision for an average of 10-11 days. Before fasting began, their diet was only fruit and vegetables.

The results of the study showed that the average reduction was 37/13. In addition, 42 of the participants followed for 27 weeks after fasting, which showed that the average blood pressure of the group was stable at 123/77.

In a previous study moderately obese women, with high blood pressure within the limits, experienced a rapid reduction in blood pressure in the first 48 hours of fasting.

Although the above studies took into account a more strict fasting protocol than intermittent fasting, I have reason to believe that intermittent fasting performed consistently and accompanied by a well-balanced diet can produce very similar results. We can say that its effects are stretched over time, but precisely the fact of not having to totally deprive yourself of food makes it easier to follow. We do not necessarily have to give up the pleasure of eating, but rather create a strategy for when to enjoy it.

ALLEVIATE OXIDATIVE STRESS AND INFLAMMATION

Before talking to you about the effects of fasting, I want to clarify how inflammatory states are created. Disease or inflammation is often thought of as something that comes to us from the outside. In reality, every disease originates within us and inflammation is a natural reaction of the body. Inflammation is often associated with pain and that pain has a very important function: to signal to us that something is wrong, a signal that the body sends us to indicate that we must act. Unfortunately, we often tend to rely on medicine that can relieve the symptom, which is the pain. Once the pain subsides we feel better and believe that we have solved the problem. The reality is that we have only eliminated the symptom, and now I will explain why.

- Inflammatory states are mainly caused by the bad habits that lead us to accumulate toxins in the body. These toxins are deposited in the tissues or organs giving rise to inflammation.

- The first bad habit is to eat excessive quantities of food or poor quality foods; these pollute the body and clog it. If the food is not adequate it will not help our regular bowel function. If the intestine is not functioning properly, many toxins remain trapped inside us.

- Sedentary life and spending little to no time outdoors make the situation worse: we are made to breathe deeply and obtaining as much vitamin D from the sun's rays as possible.

- A very important role is played in breathing: breathing deeply and with a regular rhythm (a great example for this are the breathing exercises in yoga) which allow you to bring more oxygen into the blood and get rid of excess toxins.

- Finally, we have the fast pace of life that we live in, always in a hurry, which now characterizes our civilization. Besides a physical body, we are spiritual beings who need a calm and relaxing environment for our personal well-being and state of mind. One time, I read a phrase that stuck with me "haste takes away man's dignity". This does not mean that we have to spend entire days doing nothing, but neither do we have to do everything in a rush every day of our life, following our strict schedules. This type of stress most certainly will contribute to activating an oxidative process within our system.

Oxidative stress is when the body has an imbalance of antioxidants as well as free radicals. This imbalance can cause both tissue and cell damage in overweight as well as aging people. It can also lead to various chronic illnesses like cancer, heart disease, diabetes, and has an impact on the signs of aging. Oxidative stress can trigger the inflammation that causes these diseases.

Intermittent fasting can provide your system with a reboot, that helps alleviate oxidative stress and inflammation. It also significantly reduces the risk of oxidative stress and inflammation for those overweight or obese.

During fasting, the level of zinc in the blood rises. Zinc is an element that promotes cell growth, and the healing of tissues. Zinc also facilitates the transport of oxygen into the blood, with a positive effect on the formation of collagen and therefore a better appearance of the skin.

THERAPEUTIC BENEFITS

As we have said so far and supported by many different studies, fasting and intermittent fasting allow our metabolism to eliminate toxins, damaged cells, and excess fats. All this forces the body to cell renewal. Such renewal does not simply affect the single diseases that we have seen so far in detail, but brings a general improvement in the state of health of our body. The thinner blood, the elimination of toxins, the restored intestinal function will have effects of no secondary importance on our psycho-emotional state.

Psychobiotic is a term recently coined and refers to the relationship between mind, bacteria, and intestines. In the last 10-15 years the direct connection between the intestine and the brain has been proved with certainty, so much that the intestine is said to be our "second brain". But it had been several decades since researchers began to direct their studies on the relationships between the intestinal flora and our physical and mental health.

From birth, the human organism is inhabited by a wide range of microorganisms (bacteria, fungi, protozoa, and viruses) that live and colonize exposed body surfaces, mucous membranes, and all the digestive tract, where they perform their main functions. This set of microorganisms, formerly called "intestinal flora" has recently been called microbiota.

This large community of intestinal microorganisms can produce substances that are greatly beneficial to our health. Not only the vitamins or molecules but also neurotransmitters, which, reach the brain, can generate different feelings and emotions. This is done through neurotransmitters: some microbes can produce some of the most important brain neurotransmitters. In particular, 90% of our serotonin (a neurotransmitter that controls mood, cognition, reward, learning, and memory) is synthesized in the intestine. So today we can say that the state of our intestines affects not only our general health but also our mood and mental health.

So, going back to fasting, it should not be hard for us to understand that if this helps the microbiota clean up excess toxins by making it more efficient, our body and our mind will benefit, regardless of the type of pathology, we suffer from or even if we do not have any. Whatever our starting condition is, fasting will only be of benefit to us. In other words, we can state that fasting will increase the potential for being healthier.

The disease arises from an imbalance of the microbiota, and intermittent fasting or fasting, will give the intestine a break, so it can dedicate itself to re-balance the microbiota.

This practice also has a spiritual value, as it's widely practiced for religious purposes worldwide. Although fasting is regarded as penance by some practitioners, it's also a practice of purifying your body and soul (according to the religious approach).

CHAPTER 2
FASTING FOR WOMEN OVER 50

Being a woman is one thing. Being a woman over the age of 50 is another. With age, your body begins to experience some changes. If you are self-aware, you will notice these changes early and can start working on ways to combat any of them that will interfere with your health.

Menopause indicates the period in which a woman completely ceases the reproductive cycle: after about 40 years of menstrual cycles, the cycle initially becomes irregular until it stops completely. The average age at which a woman goes through menopause is around 51 years. From this point on, the ovaries gradually stop producing estrogen hormones. In particular, the decrease in estrogen and progesterone, in turn, leads to a decrease in thyroid activity, and we know that one of the tasks of the thyroid is to control body metabolism.

The absence of estrogen causes symptoms of various severity: hot flashes, sweating, atrophy of the genitals and udder, vaginal dryness, osteoporosis, irritability, depression and sleep disturbances,

Although those described are effects of no small importance, certainly one of the side effects of menopause that puts us, women, in more difficulty is weight gain and the intimate and sometimes painful awareness that we are not young anymore. Now we have new issues to deal with. Our facial skin is changing, as is our body. We feel a little disoriented and feel the extreme need to find a new balance.

Weight gain, at this stage, is mainly due to a slowdown in "basal metabolism," that is, the number of calories consumed per day, by the resting organism, for the sole purpose of keeping vital functions active.

With age, this value tends to decrease, and you need fewer daily calories. This is why even if we have not changed our eating habits and continue to eat the same foods, we will tend to gain weight. Often, however, even reducing nutrition, there is a risk of accumulating adipose tissue, especially around the waist and abdomen and muscle mass could decrease. This leads to a problem not only aesthetic, but also of health. In fact, we become more at risk of developing certain age-related diseases. Some of the changes in your body might be subtle, but they are veiled threats to a fully functional body system and definitely to the longevity we all seek.

This is why it is imperative to seek out measures, lifestyles, and diets that could help lose fat, especially dangerous belly fat. Losing fat will drastically reduce the risks of developing health issues, such as diabetes, heart attack, and cancer. It could happen that discovering all the changes that are taking place in our bodies can leave us a little disoriented or scared. The purpose of this book is precisely not to make you feel alone or misunderstood, but to accompany you in this discovery and give you useful tools to be able to approach this phase of life with serenity and new awareness. In fact, knowing new notions and techniques is also a process of personal growth. At the same time, we could help other women in our own situation to embrace this phase with greater peace of mind. It is essential to keep your self-esteem high and the desire to always improve yourself. At 50 we are still young, we still have many years to enjoy life, make new experiences, achieve new goals! I like to consider the age of 50 as a new beginning full of opportunity.

So are you ready to find out how intermittent fasting can help us get back in shape and improve the quality of our lives?

WEIGHT LOSS

Probably the main reason that drives many women, and perhaps you too, to consider the practice of intermittent fasting is precisely weight loss. Those extra pounds make us feel uncomfortable and insecure, undermining our self-esteem and sometimes compromising our relationships with others. I support your choice to want to dig deeper into this topic in order to rediscover physical well-being. When you get to this point, you will realize that this is just one of the many advantages that intermittent fasting can offer.

My invitation, however, remains to seek in addition to physical form a type of general well-being, in which you not only see yourself well, but you feel well, in body and mind.

Once that's clear, which is essential to me, let's see how intermittent fasting will help eliminate the extra pounds.

When people have belly fat, it can cause many health problems that are associated with various diseases as it indicates a person has visceral fat. Visceral fat is fat that goes deep into the abdominal area surrounding the organs. Belly fat is terribly hard to get rid of, especially for an aging woman. Intermittent fasting has been known to help reduce not only weight but inches of over five percent of body fat in around twenty-two to twenty-five weeks (Barna, 2019).

Body fat is how the body stores energy (calories). When we don't eat anything, the body modifies several processes to make stored energy more accessible. There are changes in the activity of the nervous system and in the level of specific hormones.

- Human Growth Hormone (GH): Levels of growth hormone during a fast can increase up to 5 times. Growth hormone helps muscle growth but also fat loss

- Insulin: insulin (a hormone produced by the pancreas) increases when we eat. If we fast, it's drastically reduced. Lower insulin levels facilitate fat burning.

- Norepinephrine (it is a neurotransmitter): the nervous system sends norepinephrine to fat cells; this allows you to reduce body fat into free fatty acids that can be burned to produce energy.

Another one of the main reasons why intermittent fasting causes weight loss is due solely to the simple fact that we consume fewer calories. Since the protocols call for the "skipping" of meals during fasting periods, the calorie consumption per day will be lower.

In examining the rate of weight loss, people lost about 1 lb per week with intermittent fasting, but 2,5 lb per week with fasting every other day.

On average, people subjected to intermittent fasting show losses between 4% and 7% of their waist circumference. These results are very impressive and show that intermittent fasting can be a useful approach to lose weight.

In the review of a study, it was concluded that intermittent calorie restriction caused weight loss similar to continuous calorie restriction, yet the reduction in muscle mass was much smaller. So we can say that intermittent fasting can be useful for maintaining muscle while losing body fat. This is excellent news, considering that many diets have the disadvantage of reducing muscle mass.

MEDICAL BENEFITS

HELP TO PREVENT CANCER

Women over 50 are at a higher risk of developing some type of cancer. Intermittent fasting, as shown in research, can cut off some of the pathways that lead to cancer. Intermittent fasting can also help slow down the rate at which an existing tumor grows in the body. In fact, scientists have found that prolonged fasting also reduces the enzyme PKA, which is a hormone linked to aging. In all fairness, however, it must be said that these effects were detected by Dr. Longo's team in fasts lasting at least 72 hours and often repeated cyclically. Although not closely related to intermittent fasting, it still seemed a noteworthy fact to mention.

BREAST CANCER RECURRENCE PREVENTION

The probability of breast cancer is particularly high in overweight women going through menopause. It is estimated that 1 in 8 women develop breast cancer in their lives.

Nicholas Webster, Ph.D., a Prof. At the UC San Diego School of Medicine and senior at the VASDSH, conducted studies published in the January 25, 2021 edition of Nature Communications, on the effects of intermittent fasting. The study considered female mice with hormonal conditions comparable to post-menopause to investigate whether intermittent fasting in obese mice affected tumor development and growth and reduced metastases of lung cancer. The mice were divided into two groups: a group had access to food 24 hours a day. A second had access to food for eight hours at night when mice are more active and a third group followed an unrestricted low-fat diet. Data showed that obese mice developed high insulin levels, causing the tumor to grow rapidly. While mice that were intermittently fasting, then with a more limited diet, had the lowest insulin levels. So the studies suggest that lower insulin levels may have an anti-tumor effect.

An extended fasting period is another technique used to decrease cancer growth recurrence in breast tissue. A research study with breast cancer survivors found that the women who fasted for longer than 13 hours per night had a significant 36% lower chance of recurrence than the women who fasted for less than 13 hours per night.

LOWER RISK OF DEVELOPING TYPE 2 DIABETES

Type 2 diabetes frequently occurs in people over the age of 45. The Centers for Disease Control and Prevention report that more than 30 million Americans have diabetes (around 1 out of 10), and 90%-95% have type 2 diabetes. Type 2 diabetes can occur when your cells do not react properly to insulin. Insulin is a hormone secreted in the intestine by the pancreas, which permits cells to assimilate and utilize glucose (sugar) as energy. An impressive number of studies have shown the reduction of insulin resistance in patients that follow an intermittent fasting diet. It is best to consult with your doctor if this is applicable to you.

A study, published in the journal Cell Metabolism, evaluated the effects of intermittent fasting on a small group of people with metabolic syndrome (which involves insulin resistance) and other factors such as obesity, high blood pressure, high-fat levels (cholesterol, triglycerides), and high risk of type 2 diabetes and cardiovascular disease.

The participants, mostly obese, went through an intermittent fast for 12 weeks, consuming food for 10 hours a day (the first meal between 8 am and 10 am, the last one being between 6 pm and 8 pm) with fasting for the rest of the day, without any indication to reduce caloric intake or change the level of physical activity. At the end of the 3 months, the participants lost an average of 8 pounds, with a reduction in body fat, visceral fat, and waist circumference. Positive effects such as reduction of blood pressure and total cholesterol were also found. Eleven participants had a form of pre-diabetes and one participant type 2 diabetes: in this subgroup, intermittent fasting led to a reduction in blood sugar and glided hemoglobin.

The study concludes that a regular cycle of nutrition and fasting could be an effective strategy in treating metabolic syndrome and thus reducing the risk of type 2 diabetes and cardiovascular diseases associated with it.

IMPROVED HEART HEALTH

When it comes to heart health, we mainly consider triglycerides, cholesterol, and blood pressure. As suggested by the above study fasting can reduce them, improving the resting heart rate. Unfortunately, our society suffers from overfeeding, we eat too much and foods are too rich in fat, sugar, and protein. They are all fundamental nutrients but only if taken in the right amount. When there is an excess they make the blood thicker, resulting in the clogging of the blood vessels creating heart problems.

But not only the amount of food we consume and its quality determine the viscosity of the blood. Packaged foods, fast foods, ready to eat meals are very rich in sugars, fats, and preservatives. Any of these eaten frequently will result in a very negative impact on the fluidity of our blood.

OSTEOARTHRITIS

Osteoarthritis is a widespread pathology, which mainly affects menopausal women. After the age of 50, the main trigger is the estrogen deficiency caused by exhaustion of ovarian activity.

It is an inflammation at the level of the joint that manifests itself by swelling, pain, and stiffness.

Periodic dietary restrictions have the potential to deactivate the inflammatory state. Some of the researchers discovered that the fasting period in fact affects the way the body produces hormones. This will help strengthen the bones and forestall against things like arthritic symptoms and lower back pain.

OTHER BENEFITS

ANTI-AGING PROCESS

Certainly being 50 today is not the same as having 50 a few decades ago. Given the increased average of life span, the many stimuli that life offers us, the greater opportunities and new paths of personal growth, the modern-day lifestyle includes too much stress, work commitments, frenetic rhythms and often there is no time to take care of oneself and one's diet with serenity. Whether we like it or not, these factors contribute to the aging process.

You are probably wondering what intermittent fasting can do to slow down this process, or if that is even possible. Intermittent fasting is not "the fountain of youth," and it will not grant you immortality. However, it can still l reduce oxidative damage. The fasting body is dedicated to renewal. Furthermore, fasting accelerates the cleaning of blood vessels, cells, and the environment in which they swim. Non-recyclable toxins are eliminated and new ones are produced that repair all biological functions, including the cells of the skin and all the tissues present in the body. In short, fasting is an intensive session of body repair and purification thus balances the overload of modern life. These will all make you feel and look younger, fresher and will extend life expectancy.

BETTER MENTAL PERFORMANCE

Menopause affects not only physical factors, but often also those of a psycho-affective nature such as irritability, unstable mood, fatigue, anxiety, depression, impaired concentration, and memory, decreased sexual desire.

A few paragraphs ago I told you about the intestinal microbiota understood as the set of bacteria that populate our intestine and determine our health. We have seen how a healthy microbiota also affects the state of the brain. The crucial role of the microbiota in brain development was demonstrated in an animal study. It was found that mice raised in sterile (free of bacteria) environments exhibited alterations of the nervous system and exaggerated physiological reactions to stress. Surprisingly, if their intestines were recolonized with bacteria (through probiotics) the central nervous system improved considerably.

Our microbiota tends to change its composition according to various environmental factors such as lifestyle, the use of drugs and antibiotics, and the intake of foods with low fiber content. Diet is considered to be among the main factors that impact the human gut microbiota throughout the life span. Probiotics (live micro-organisms) administered in adequate quantities are believed to benefit our microbiota. A 2015 article cites 5 clinical trials in which participants had undergone treatment with probiotics. The result was that these reduced the risk of developing depression in healthy people and that they relieved symptoms of depression in those who already had it.

The discovery of the microbiota and its relationship with the brain allows us to open new frontiers for medicine. We now know that the intestine behaves like a huge sensory organ, constantly feeding the brain with information.

After this necessary premise on the role of the microbiota, we can analyze how also in this case intermittent fasting can be of great benefit. Intermittent fasting enhances cognitive function and also is very useful when it comes to boosting your brainpower. There are several factors of intermittent fasting which can support this claim. First of all, it increases the level of brain-derived neurotrophic factor (also known as BDNF), a protein in your brain that can interact with the parts of your brain responsible for controlling cognitive and memory functions as well as learning. BDNF can even protect and stimulate the growth of new brain cells. Through IF, you will enter the ketogenic state, during which your body turns fat into energy, by using ketones. Ketones can also feed your brain, and therefore improve your mental acuity, productivity, and energy.

HELPS WITH SLEEP AND CLARITY

Sleep disorders affect the amount of time we are able to devote to sleep, but also the quality of the latter. Science affirms that those who suffer from sleep problems have multiple consequences that in the long run affect our psycho-physical well-being. Sleep is essential as it allows the body to recover and regenerate, completing the normal detoxification tasks.

Hormonal changes in the body can cause one's sleeping pattern to be destabilized, especially around post-menstrual age. Many older women have testified how the intermittent fasting lifestyle has improved their sleeping patterns. With fasting and intermittent fasting, attention, concentration, and memory can greatly improve as well as logical and intuitive skills. This cognitive well-being does not act so much on the duration of the hours of sleep, but on its quality. Sleep is more serene and restful and the need for sleep decreases.

BOOSTS PRODUCTIVITY

Now that you learned that the microbiota and the brain are closely interconnected, you can better understand how a healthy intestinal environment affects our cognitive faculties. You also discovered that fasting promotes cell renewal.

So the microbiota after a fast or a period of intermittent fasting is noticeably re-balanced. The effect will be extraordinary lucidity. The vital energies are strengthened, original solutions are found to practical or existential problems, initiatives and programs are planned for the future. In other words, you feel better, more active, and confident about the future.

CHAPTER 3
HOW TO PRACTICE FASTING

INTERMITTENT FASTING PROTOCOLS

There are so many different ways to practice intermittent fasting. I will guide you through 10 specific and different methods for IF before finishing with a section on how to make your choice. At the end of this chapter, if you have chosen to test the IF, you should feel that your IF plans have direction and form, and you should be excited to implement these new plans in your daily routine.

EXPLANATION OF DIFFERENT METHODS

Before you can start intermittent fasting and incorporate it into your lifestyle, you must know all the possibilities to choose the right one for you, your goals, your habits, and your body/personality type. Read the following ten tips to discover which methods seem most appropriate.

LEAN GAIN METHOD

The method of lean gain essentially focuses on the combined efforts of rigorous exercise, fasting, and a healthy diet. The fame surrounding this approach comes from its acclaimed success in converting fat directly into muscle. The goal is to fast every day for 14-16 hours, starting from waking up.

The ideal approach to lean gains seems to be to get up and fast until 1:00 pm, stretch, and warm up before training just before noon. Starting at noon, you would start training in any exercise you choose for an hour or less, and you will end up breaking quickly around 1 pm. Your meal at this time would be the best of the day. You attended your days as always in the past and, as far as possible, return to eat around 4 pm, then eat for the last time around 9 pm. If you choose this approach and feel a little overwhelmed, you can work up to 15 hours, starting with 13 or 14 hours of fasting only during the first week.

LEAN GAIN PROTOCOL	FAST	LUNCH	DINNER	FAST
Monday				
Thuesday				
Wednesday				
Thursday				
Friday				
Saturday				
Sunday				
	0 PM/ 12 PM	12 AM	8 PM	8 PM/ 0 AM

METHOD 16:8

The 16:8 method is one of the most popular among the fasters. You spend 16 hours on an empty stomach every day, and the other 8 hours are your window to eat. Many people try to choose the 8-hour feeding period as the time when they are most active. If you are a night person, do not hesitate to do it a little later. Stop eating during the day as much as possible and then have breakfast around 3 or 4 in the afternoon. For people who have breakfast early in the morning, for example, around 11 am, or lunch from 7 pm to 4 a.m. It is an incredibly flexible method that works for many different types of people. It is also flexible when you decide to try a particular fast food relationship. For example, if you don't seem to be playing with the food window from 11 a.m. to 7 p.m., you can change the next day to meet your needs better. You can try to wait until later for breakfast! Try what you need to do, as long as you keep that ratio of 16:8 hours. While the lean gain method technically applies the same hourly rate, it is much more rigorous than a healthy diet and exercise regime. The 16:8 method does not need any exercise reinforcement, but it depends on the professional. It is always better to try to add healthy dietary options to your IF feeding schedule, but do not try to limit too many calories, as it may cause dizziness and low energy. With 16:8, you can eat what you need and exchange the hours you want.

16 : 8 PROTOCOL	FAST	FEED	FEED	FAST
Monday				
Thuesday				
Wednesday				
Thursday				
Friday				
Saturday				
Sunday				
	0 AM/ 10 PM	10 PM/ 4 PM	4 PM/ 6 PM	6 PM/ 0 AM

METHOD 14:10

Similar to method 16:8, 14:10 requires fasting and feeding on multiple levels every day. In this case, I would fast for 14 hours and then eat for 10 hours. This method has the same flexibility of 16:8 in terms of what time of day it is organized and how easy it is to solve problems. But it is also flexible in the sense that the window for eating lasts two hours long, it can accommodate people with more intense physical routines or daily needs, as well as people who need to eat a little later during the day.

14:10 PROTOCOL	FAST	FEED	FEED	FAST
Monday				
Thuesday				
Wednesday				
Thursday				
Friday				
Saturday				
Sunday				
	0 AM/ 8 AM	8 AM /4 PM	4 PM/ 6 PM	6 PM / 0 AM

METHOD 20:4

While the 14:10 method was a simpler step than the 16:8 method, the 20:4 method is a step forward in terms of difficulty. Without a doubt, it is a more intense method, since it requires 20 hours of fasting every day with only a 4-hour feeding period for the individual to obtain all their nutrients and energy. Many people who try this method end up eating a large meal with several snacks or two smaller meals with fewer snacks. The 20:4 method is flexible in the sense where the individual chooses how the window for eating is divided between meals and snacks.

The 20:4 method is complicated since many people instinctively eat excessively during the feeding window, but it is neither necessary nor healthy. People who choose the 20:4 method should try to keep portions of food the same size they normally would without fasting. Experiencing how many snacks are needed will also be useful in this method. Many people end up working up to 20:4 with other methods, depending on what their bodies are capable of handling and what they are ready to try. Few begin with 20:4, so if it doesn't work right away, don't be too hard on yourself! Return to 16:8 and then see how soon you can return to where you want to be.

20:4 PROTOCOL	FAST	FEED	FAST	FAST
Monday				
Thuesday				
Wednesday				
Thursday				
Friday				
Saturday				
Sunday				
	8 AM / 2PM	2 PM / 6PM	6 PM / 8 PM	8 PM / 00 AM

THE WARRIOR METHOD

The warrior's method is quite similar to the 20:4 method in which the individual fasts for 20 hours a day and stops quickly for a period of 4 hours to eat. However, the difference lies in the perspective and mentality of the professional. The thought process behind the warrior's method is that in ancient times, the hunter who returned home from stalking prey or the warrior who returned home from the battle only received one meal a day.

A meal should provide sustenance for the rest of the day, recovering energy for the future. Therefore, warrior method professionals are advised to eat an excellent meal when they have breakfast and that the meal should be rich in fat, protein, and carbohydrates for the rest of the day (and for the days to come). However, as with the 20:4 method, it can sometimes be too intense for professionals, and it is very easy to reduce it a lot by inventing a method like 18:6 or 17:7. If it doesn't work, don't force it, but try to do it for a week to see if the problem is your stubbornness or if it is just a coincidence with the method.

20:4 PROTOCOL	SMALL AMOUNT OF FRUIT OR VEGETABLES	SMALL AMOUNT OF FRUIT OR VEGETABLES	LARGE MEAL	SMALL AMOUNT OF FRUIT OR VEGETABLES	FAST
Monday					
Thuesday					
Wednesday					
Thursday					
Friday					
Saturday					
Sunday					
	8 AM / 12 PM	12 PM/ 4 PM	4	4 PM / 8 PM	8PM/ 8 AM

12:12 METHOD

The 12:12 method is somewhat simpler, along with the lines of 14:10, instead of 16:8 or 20:4. Beginners in intermittent fasting would do well to try immediately. Some people sleep 12 hours every night and can easily wake up from the fasting period, ready to join the window to eat. Many people use this method in their lives without even knowing it. However, to follow the 12:12 method in your life, you will want to be as determined as possible. Be sure to be strict with the limits of 12 hours. Make sure it works and feels good in your body, so we invite you to improve things and try, for example, 14:10 or maybe your invention, like 15:11. As always, start with what works and then go up (or down) to what makes you feel good (and maybe even better).

12:12 PROTOCOL	FAST	FEED	FEED	FAST
Monday				
Thuesday				
Wednesday				
Thursday				
Friday				
Saturday				
Sunday				
	0 AM/08 AM	8 AM / 12 PM	12 PM/ 8 PM	8 PM/ 0 AM

5:2 METHOD

The 5:2 method is popular among those who wish to improve things in general. Instead of fasting and eating every day, these people practice fasting two full days a week. The other five days are free to eat, exercise or diet, but the other two days (which can be consecutive or scattered during the week) must be strictly fasting days. However, for those fasting days, it is not as if the individual cannot eat anything at all. It is allowed to consume no more than 500 calories per day for this intermittent fasting method. I suppose that these days of fasting would be better known as "limited hiring" days, as it is a more precise description. The 5:2 method is extremely rewarding, but it is also one of the most difficult to try. If you have problems with this method, do not be afraid to experiment next week with a method like 14:10 or 16:8, where you fast and eat every day. If this works best for you, stick with it! However, if you have "active" days and "free" days with fasting and feeding, there are also other alternatives.

5: 2 PROTOCOL				
Monday				
Thuesday		ONLY	500	KCAL
Wednesday				
Thursday				
Friday				
Saturday		ONLY	500	KCAL
Sunday				
	00 AM/08 AM	8 AM / 12 PM	12 PM / 8 PM	8 PM / 00 AM

EAT-STOP-EAT METHOD (24 HOURS)

The method to stop eating for 24 hours is another option for people who want to have "on" and "free" days between fasting and eating. It is a little less intense than the 5:2 method and is much more flexible for the individual, depending on what he needs. For example, if you need a 24-hour literal fast every week and that's it, you can do it. On the other hand, if you want something more flexible than the type of 5:2 method to happen, you can work with what you want and create a method that surrounds those desires and goals. The most successful approaches to the Eat-Stop-Eat method involved a more rigorous diet (or at least a prudent and healthy diet) during the 5 or 6 days in which the individual participates in the free meal window of the week. For the individual to see success with weight loss, there will also have to be a caloric restriction (or a high nutrition approach) for those 5 or 6 days, so that the body has a version of consistency in the health content and nutrition. In the one or two days a week that the individual decides to fast, there may still be a very limited calorie intake. As with the 5:2 method, during these fasting days, you cannot consume more than 500 calories in food and beverages so that the body can maintain the flow of energy and more.

If the individual exercises, those training days must be reserved for 5 or 6 days of free food. The same applies to method 5:2. Try not to exercise (at least not in excess) on the days chosen to fast. Your body will not appreciate the additional stress when you eat so few calories. As always, you can choose to switch from Eat-Stop-Eat to another method if it works easily, and you are interested in something else. Also, you can start with a rigorous 24-hour method and then move on to a more flexible Eat-Stop-Eat approach. Do what you think is right and never be afraid to solve one method simply by choosing another.

EAT STOP EAT				
Monday				
Thuesday	FAST 24 H			
Wednesday				
Thursday				
Friday				
Saturday	FAST 24 H			
Sunday				
	00AM/ 08AM	8 AM/ 12 PM	12 PM/ 8 PM	8 PM/ 00 AM

ALTERNATIVE DAY METHOD

The alternative day method is similar to the Eat-Stop-Eat and 5:2 method because it focuses on individual "on" and "off" days for fasting and eating. The difference for this method, in particular, is that you end up fasting at least 2 days a week and sometimes for 4 days. Some people follow very rigorous approaches to the alternate day method and fast every other day, consuming only 500 calories or less on fasting days. Some people, on the other hand, are much more flexible and tend to eat for two days, one day on an empty stomach, two days, one day on an empty stomach, etc. The alternative day method is even more flexible than getting up in that sense, since it allows the individual to choose how to alternate food and fasting, depending on what works best for the body and mind. The alternative day method is like a step up from the eat-stop-eat and 24-hour methods, especially if the individual alternates the fast of one day and the next day eating, etc. Surprisingly, this more intense style of fasting works particularly well for people who work in equally intense fitness regimes. People who consume more calories per day than 2000 (which is true for many bodybuilders and exercise enthusiasts) will have more to gain from the alternative day method since they only need to reduce their fasting diet to about 25 percent of standard caloric intake. Therefore, those fasting days can still provide solid nutritional support to fitness experts, helping them sculpt their bodies and maintain a new level of health.

ALTERNATIVE DAY FASTING				
Monday				
Thuesday	FAST 24 H			
Wednesday				
Thursday	FAST 24 H			
Friday				
Saturday	FAST 24 H			
Sunday				
	0 AM/ 08 AM	8 AM / 12 PM	12PM/8PM	8PM/0AM

SPONTANEOUS OMISSION METHOD

The alternative day method and the Eat-Stop-Eat method are certainly flexible in their approaches to when the individual fasts and when he eats. However, none of the plans mentioned above are as flexible as the method of spontaneous omission.

The spontaneous jump method requires the individual to skip meals within each day, whenever you want (and when it is perceived that the body can handle it). Many people with sensitive digestive systems or practice regimens of more intense physical conditioning will start your experience with IF through the spontaneous jump method before moving on to something more intense. People who have very messy daily schedules or people who are around food a lot but forget to eat will benefit from this method, as it works well with chaotic schedules and unplanned energies. Despite this chaotic and disorganized potential, the method of spontaneous omission can also be more structured and organized, depending on what you do about it! For example, someone who wants more structure can choose which food each day they want to skip. Suppose you choose to skip breakfast every day. Therefore, your method of spontaneous omission will be structured around you, making sure to skip breakfast (that is, do not eat at least until 12:00 p.m.) every day. Whatever you need to do to make this method work, try it! This method is made for experimentation and adventure.

SPONTANEOUS MEAL SKIPPPING	BREAKFAST	LUNCH	DINNER	FAST
Monday				
Thuesday	FAST			
Wednesday				
Thursday			FAST	
Friday				
Saturday				
Sunday		FAST		
	8 AM/ 12 PM	12 PM / 4 PM	4 PM/8PM	8PM/8AM

CRESCENDO METHOD

The last method that is worth mentioning is the crescendo method, which is very suitable for the practice of women (since high-intensity fasts can be very harmful to their anatomy). This approach is made for internal awareness, soft introductions, and gradual additions, depending on what works and what doesn't. It is a very active type of trial and error method. Through the crescendo method, the individual begins to fast only 2 or 3 days a week, and on those days of fasting, it would not be a very intense fast. It would not even be so strict that the individual should not consume more than 500 calories, as with 5:2, Eat-Stop-Eat, and others. Instead, these "fast" days would be trial periods for methods such as 12:12, 14:10, 16:8, or 20:4. The remaining 4 or 5 days of the week would be open periods for eating. The professional is encouraged to maintain a healthy diet throughout the week. The Crescendo method works extremely well for female practitioners because it allows them to see how methods like 14:10 or 12:12 will affect their bodies without attaching them to the hook, line, and plumb line of the method. It allows them to see what each method does at the hormonal level, menstrual tendency, and mood swings. Therefore, the crescendo method encourages these people to be more in touch with their bodies before moving too fast towards something that can cause serious anatomical and hormonal damage. The Crescendo method will also work very well for overweight or diabetic professionals, as it will allow them to have these same "trial period" moments with everyone.

MOST COMMON MISTAKES

When you are looking to make any significant adjustments in your life, it can take time to discover exactly how to do it in the best ways possible. Many people will make mistakes and have some setbacks as they seek to improve their health through intermittent fasting. Some of these mistakes are minor and can easily be overcome, whereas others may be dangerous and could cause serious repercussions if they are not caught in time.

In this chapter, we are going to explore common mistakes that people tend to make when they are on the intermittent fasting diet. We will also explore why these mistakes are made, and how they can be avoided. It is important that you read through this chapter before you actually commit to the diet itself. That way, you can ensure that you are avoiding any potential mistakes beforehand. This will help you in avoiding unwanted problems and achieving your results with greater success and fewer setbacks.

KEEP IN MIND:

- Food Quality: The foods you eat are important. Try to eat mostly whole grains, a wide variety of vegetables and try to reduce processed foods. I am a great supporter of fruit and vegetables, raw if possible (because they maintain their properties unaltered).

- Calories: In intermittent fasting, it is not necessary to count the calories ingested. However, we must try to eat "normally" during the non-fasting periods and we must not compensate for what we have not eaten during the fasting hours.

- Patience and Organization: The body needs time to adjust to an intermittent fasting protocol. It is recommended to be consistent with meal times. The organization is also important because we risk arriving hungry at the scheduled time if we have not prepared anything in advance. Otherwise, we run the risk of eating the first thing we find even if it's unhealthy

You should also keep this chapter handy as you embark on your intermittent fasting diet. That way, if you do begin to notice that things are not going as you had hoped, you can easily refer back to this chapter and get the information that you need to adjust your diet and improve your results.

SWITCHING TOO FAST

A significant number of people fail to comply with their new diets because they attempt to go too hard too fast. Trying to jump too quickly can result in you feeling too extreme of a departure from your normal. As a result, both psychologically and physically you are put under a significant amount of stress from your new diet. This can lead to you feeling like the diet is not actually effective and like you are suffering more than you are benefitting from it.

If you are someone who eats regularly and who snacks frequently, switching to the intermittent fasting diet will take time and patience. I cannot stress the importance of your transition period enough.

It is not uncommon to want to jump off the deep end when you are making a lifestyle change. Often, we want to expe-rience great results right away and we are excited about the switch. However, after a few days, it can feel stressful. Because you didn't give your mind and body enough time to adapt to the changes, you ditch your new diet in favor of more comfor-table things.

Fasting is something that should always be acclimated to over a period of time. There is no set period, it needs to be done based on what feels right for you and your body. If you are not properly listening to your body and it needs you are going to end up suffering in major ways. Especially with diets like intermittent fasting, letting yourself adapt to the changes and listening to your body's needs can ensure that you are not ne-glecting your body in favor of strictly following someone else guide on what to do.

CHOOSING THE WRONG PLAN FOR YOUR LIFESTYLE

It is not uncommon to forget the importance of picking a fa-sting cycle that actually fits with your lifestyle and then fit-ting it in. Trying to fast to a cycle that does not fit with your lifestyle will ultimately result in you feeling inconvenienced by your diet and struggling to maintain it.

Often, the way we naturally eat is in accordance with what we feel fits into our lifestyle in the best way possible. So, if you look at your present diet and notice that there are a lot of convenience meals and they happen all throughout the day, you can conclude two things: you are busy, and you eat when you can. Picking a diet that allows you to eat when you can is important in helping you stick to it. It is also important that you begin searching for healthier convenience options so that you can get the most out of your diet.

Anytime you make a lifestyle change, such as with your diet, you need to consider what your lifestyle actually is. In an ideal world, you may be able to adapt everything to suit your dreamy needs completely. However, in the real world, there are likely many aspects of your lifestyle that are simply not practical to adjust. Picking a diet that suits your lifestyle rather than picking a lifestyle that suits your diet makes far more sense.

Taking the time to actually document what your present eating habits are like before you embark on your intermittent fasting diet is a great way to begin. Focus on what you are already eating and how often and consider diets that will serve your lifestyle. You should also consider your activity levels and how much food you truly need at certain times of the day. For example, if you have a spin class every morning, fasting until noon might not be a good idea as you could end up hungry and exhausted after your class. Choosing the dieting pattern that fits your lifestyle will help you maintain your diet so you can continue receiving great results from it.

EATING TOO MUCH OR NOT ENOUGH

Focusing on what you are eating and how much you are eating is important. This is one of the biggest reasons why a gradual and intentional transition can be helpful. If you are used to eating throughout the entire day, attempting to eat the same amount in a shorter window can be challenging. You may find yourself feeling stuffed and far too full to actually sustain that amount of eating on a day-to-day basis. As a result, you may find yourself not eating enough.

If you are new to intermittent fasting and you take the leap too quickly, it is not unusual to find yourself scarfing down as much food as you possibly can the moment your eating window opens back up. As a result, you find yourself feeling sick, too full, and uncomfortable. Your body also struggles to process and digest that much food after having been fasting for any given period of time. This can be even harder on your body if you have been using a more intense fast and then you stuff yourself. If you find yourself doing this, it may be a sign that you have transitioned too quickly and that you need to slow down and back off.

You might also find yourself not eating enough. Attempting to eat the same amount that you typically eat in 12-16 hours in just 8-12 hours can be challenging. It may not sound so drastic on paper, but if you are not hungry you may simply not feel like eating. As a result, you may feel compelled to skip meals. This can lead to you not getting enough calories and nutrition on a daily basis. In the end, you find yourself not eating enough and feeling unsatisfied during your fasting windows.

The best way to combat this is to begin practicing making calorie-dense foods before you actually start intermittent fasting. Learning what recipes you can make and how much each meal needs to have in order to help you reach your goals is a great way to get yourself ready and show yourself what it truly takes to succeed. Then, begin gradually shortening your eating window and giving yourself the time to work up to eating enough during those eating windows without overeating. In the end, you will find yourself feeling amazing and not feeling unsatisfied or overeating as you maintain your diet.

YOUR FOOD CHOICES ARE NOT HEALTHY ENOUGH

Even if you are eating according to the keto diet or any other dietary style while you are intermittently fasting, it is not uncommon to find yourself eating the wrong food choices. Simply knowing what to eat and what to avoid is not enough. You need to spend some time getting to understand what specific vitamins, and minerals you need to thrive. That way, you can eat a diet that is rich in these specific nutrients. Then, you can trust that your body has everything that it needs to thrive on your diet.

Even though intermittent fasting does not technically outline what you should and should not eat, it is not a one-size-fits-all diet that can help you lose weight while eating anything you want. In other words, excessive amounts of junk foods will still have a negative impact on you, even if you're eating during the right windows.

It is important that you choose a diet that is going to help you maintain everything you need to function optimally. Ideally, you should combine intermittent fasting with another diet such as the keto diet, the Mediterranean diet, or any other diet that supports you in eating healthfully. Following the guidelines of these healthier diets ensures that you are incorporating the proper nutrients into your diet so that you can stay healthy.

Eating the right nutrients is essential as it will support your body in healthy hormonal balance and bodily functions. This is how you can keep your organs functioning effectively so that everything works the way it should. As a result, you end up feeling healthier and experiencing greater benefits from your diet. It is imperative that you focus on this if you want to have success with your intermittent fasting diet.

YOU ARE NOT DRINKING ENOUGH FLUIDS

Many people do not realize how much hydration their foods actually give them on a day-to-day basis. Food like fruit and vegetables are filled with hydration that supports your body in healthily functions. If you are not eating as many, then you can guarantee that you are not getting as much hydration as you need to be. This means that you need to focus on increasing your hydration levels.

When you are dehydrated you can experience many unwanted symptoms that can make intermittent fasting a challenge. Increased headaches, muscle cramping, and increased hunger are all side effects of dehydration. A great way to combat dehydration is to make sure that you keep water nearby and sip it often. At least once every fifteen minutes to half an hour you should have a good drink of water. This will ensure that you are getting plenty of fresh water into your system.

Other ways that you can maintain your hydration levels include drinking low-calorie sports drinks, bone broth, tea, and coffee. Essentially, drinking low-calorie drinks throughout the course of the entire day can be extremely helpful in supporting your health. Make sure that you do not exceed your fasting calorie maximum, however, or you will stop gaining the benefits of fasting. As well, water should always be your first choice above any other drinks to maintain your hydration. However, including some of the others from time to time can support you and keep things interesting so that you can stay hydrated but not bored.

If you begin to experience any symptoms of dehydration, make sure that you immediately begin increasing the amount of water that you are drinking. Dehydration can lead to far more serious side effects beyond headaches and muscle cramps if you are not careful. If you find that you are prone to not drinking enough water on a daily basis, consider setting a reminder on your phone that keeps you drinking plenty throughout the day.

The best way to tell that you are staying hydrated enough is to pay attention to how frequently you are peeing. If you are staying in a healthy range of hydration, you should be peeing at least once every single hour. If you aren't, this means that you need to be drinking more water, even if you aren't experiencing any side effects of dehydration. Typically, if you have already begun experiencing side effects then you have waited too long. You want to maintain healthy hydration without waiting for symptoms like headaches and muscle aches to inform you that it is time to start drinking more. This ensures that your body stays happy and healthy and that you are not causing unnecessary suffering or stress to your body throughout the day.

YOU ARE GIVING UP TOO QUICKLY

A lot of people assume that eating the intermittent fasting diet means that they will see the benefits of their eating habits immediately. This is not the case. While intermittent fasting does typically offer great results fairly quickly, it does take some time for these results to begin appearing. The exact amount of time depends on many factors. How long it has taken you to transition, what and how you are eating during eating windows, and how much activity you are getting throughout the day all contribute to your results.

You might feel compelled to quickly give up if you do not begin noticing your desired results right away, but trust that this is not going to help you. Some people require several weeks before they really begin seeing the benefits of their dieting. This does not mean that it is not working, it simply means that it has taken them some time to find the right balance so that they can gain their desired results and stay healthy.

If you are feeling like throwing in the towel, first take a few minutes to consider what you are doing and how it may be negatively impacting your results. A great way to do this is to try using your food diary once again. For a few days, track how you are eating in accordance with the intermittent fasting diet and what it is doing for you. Get a clear idea of how much you are eating, what you are eating, and when you are eating it. Also, track the amount of physical activity that you are doing on a daily basis.

Through tracking your food intake and exercise levels, you might find that you are not experiencing the results you desire because you are eating too much or not enough in comparison to the amount of energy you are spending each day. Then, you can easily work towards adjusting your diet to find a balance that supports you in getting everything you need and also seeing the results that you desire.

In most cases, intermittent fasting diets are not working because they are not being used right for the individual person. Although the general requirements are somewhat the same, each of us has unique needs based on our lifestyles and our unique makeup. If you are willing to invest time in finding the right balance for yourself then you can guarantee that you can overcome this and experience great results from your fasting.

YOU ARE GETTING TOO INTENSE OR PUSHING IT

If you are really focused on achieving your desired results, you might feel compelled to push your diet further than what is reasonable for you. For example, attempting to take on too intense of a fasting cycle or trying to do more than your body can reasonably handle. It is not uncommon for people to try and push themselves beyond reasonable measures to achieve their desired results. Unfortunately, this rarely results in them achieving what they actually set out to achieve. It can also have severe consequences.

At the end of the day, listening to your body and paying attention to exactly what it needs is important. You need to be taking care of yourself through proper nutrition and proper exercise levels. You also need to balance these two in a way that serves your body, rather than in a way that leads to you feeling sick and unwell. If you push your body too far, the negative consequences can be severe and long-lasting. In some cases, they may even be life-threatening.

In some cases, pushing your body to a certain extent is necessary. For example, if you are seeking to build more muscle then you want to push yourself to work out enough that your workouts are actually effective. However, if you are pushing yourself to the point that you are beginning to experience negative side effects from your diet, you need to drawback. While certain amounts of side effects are fairly normal early on, experiencing intense side effects, having side effects that don't go away, or having them return is not good. You want to work towards maintaining and minimizing your side effects, not constantly living alongside them. After all, what is the point of adjusting your diet and lifestyle to serve your health if you are not actually feeling healthy while you do it?

Make sure that you check in with yourself on a daily basis to see to it that your physical needs are being met. That way, if anything begins to feel excessive or any symptoms begin to increase, you can focus on minimizing or eliminating them right away. Paying close attention to your needs and looking at your goals long-term rather than trying to reach them immediately is the best way to ensure that you reach your health goals without actually compromising your health while attempting to do so. In the end, you will feel much better about doing it this way.

CHAPTER 4
PRACTICAL SUPPORT TO FASTING

THE RIGHT MINDSET

We all know in the 21st century that well-being starts with healthy eating habits. Then why is it so difficult to stick to a balanced diet? The grocery store's aisles, posters on the doctor's offices, and even some TV advertisements use vivid colors and bold lettering to advertise healthy living. Women over 50 years are especially advised to watch what they eat as it is easier for them to gain weight than lose it.

The issue is not because people don't want to change their eating habits; it's that they don't even know how to do it. They get on board a new weight-loss plan, which they soon discard as such diets are often unsustainable when compared with regular lifestyles.

That's not the best way to go for a balanced lifestyle. Instead, you want to make a meaningful, permanent improvement, but you have to make sure you are doing it right. The guide below will help and show you how to stick to healthy eating habits. By setting realistic expectations and being persistent, you will find that good eating patterns are now well within your grasp even though they were impossible in the past. Each diet and weight-loss plan has its benefits and drawbacks, so you have to prepare your mind for it if you want to succeed.

The hardest factor in weight loss is changing your attitude about how to lose weight.

Many people attempt to lose weight with the worst imaginable mental state. They bolt into diets and workout programs out of personal deprecation, all the while squeezing their "trouble" spots, branding themselves "fat" and feeling entirely less than that. They get distracted with results, rely on fast solutions, and lose sight of what good health is all about.

This kind of thought can be harmful. Instead of concentrating on the benefits that can come from weight loss — such as improved well-being, healthier life, greater satisfaction of daily lives, and the avoidance of diabetes and cardiac disease — these people focus on their pessimistic feelings. Eventually, poor thinking leads to disappointment.

Changing your mentality about weight loss goes beyond feeling good; it's about the outcome. A study at the University of Syracuse indicates that the more unhappy women are with their bodies, the more likely they are to skip exercise. And just focusing on the fact that you're overweight is forecasting a potential weight gain – according to studies reported in the International Journal of Obesity in 2015.

Although psychologists emphasize that your actions are determined by how you view yourself and your core personality (seeing yourself as being overweight or undesirable makes you behave accordingly), genetics may also play a role. A study published in Psychosomatic Medicine journal also suggested that cortisol, the stress hormone, is secreted by the adrenal glands every time you get yourself down or think about your weight, which further causes weight gain.

IT ALL STARTS WITH YOUR MINDSET

The problem with a lot of trendy diets is that they don't want you to think differently. They tell you to make a drastic adjustment to your eating habits. This is not healthy. If you are actively trying to change your eating habits, then first you have to fix your way of thinking about food.

Many people who are struggling to eat healthily have what researchers term a "closed mentality." These people believe that nothing can ever change, and they take this belief with them in beginning a new weight loss plan. They think that their health issues are simply the effects of poor biology, or that the embarrassment of solving the problem would reverse any improvements.

For certain people with a fixed mentality, long before it begins, a change of diet is futile. In reality, many would prefer to stay obese because it feels safer and less stressful than attempting to make a change in lifestyle.

Unfortunately, anyone who wants to move to a healthier lifestyle without changing their attitude first will soon get discouraged. That's because the journey to a healthy lifestyle doesn't happen overnight. There are no magic foods, no matter what the magazine said or what some star did to shed baby weight or to dress for a new role. If you are someone with a fixed mindset starting a weight loss diet, you'll undoubtedly come to think the plan failed when you don't see any significant difference — reinforcing your original fears. The diet's failure will only make it harder for you to begin a new journey to eating healthy. There is another mindset that Psychologists refer to as a "growth mindset." While the fixed mindset believes little else can be changed, the growth mindset thinks things are continually evolving.

People with a growth mindset don't design their thoughts to be negative. Instead, they understand that small mistakes are just part of improvement. They realize that risks are only a minor problem in achieving something big. Therefore, people with a growth mindset recognize that progress needs incremental steps in the right direction, rather than resigning themselves to the inevitable.

What kind of attitude do you have? If you have a fixed mindset, how do you make the necessary change?

One of the easiest ways to begin making a change is by collecting information about the process. I highly recommend that you maintain a journal. This is so when you see subtle improvements leading up to a significant transition, they don't get lost. Start by writing down your expectations and record whether or not you have successfully met them.

A growth mindset is not a crazy dreamer mindset when it comes to goals. When setting your targets, always make sure that they are fair. Keep note of how many balanced meals you consume, relative to how many might not be. Act to increase the number of nutritious meals you consume each week.

You've got to understand more than anything that your mindset may be what held you off. The good news is that you're well on your way to make a meaningful difference when you know that mindset is part of the problem!

Below are some steps you can take to change your mindset.

- **ADJUST YOUR PRIORITIES**

The reason might be to lose weight, but that should not be the target. Instead, the objectives should be small, manageable stuff that you have full power to control. Have you consumed five fruit and veggie servings today? That's one goal achieved. What about 8 hours of sleep; have you got them in? If so, you can cross them off your list.

- **GRAVITATE TO POSITIVITY**

It is vital to Surround yourself with the Good. Doing so offers you a relaxing, socially healthy environment to invest in yourself. Don't be afraid to ask for help or support.

- **RETHINK PUNISHMENTS AND REWARDS**

Remember that making healthier decisions is a way to practice self-care. Food is not a reward, and a workout is not a penalty. They are all necessary to take care of your body and to make you do the best you can. You deserve both.

Taking a few minutes at the start of your exercise or at the beginning of your day to calm down, and simply concentrate on breathing will help you set your goals, communicate with your body, and even reduce the stress response of your body.

Find a quiet space wherever you are (even at work), and try this exercise to help you feel more relaxed and ready to tackle the rest of your day. Lie with your legs outstretched on your back and put one hand on your stomach and one on your shoulder. Breathe in for four seconds through your nose, stay for two, and exhale for six seconds through your lips. Repeat this process for 5-10 minutes, focusing on the sensation of your stomach rising and falling with each breath.

- **24 HOUR GOALS**

Having patience is essential when you are losing weight. Plus, if you concentrate on reaching genuinely reachable targets, such as taking 10.000 steps each day, you don't need to be caught up in your list of goals. New accomplishments come in every 24 hours; concentrate on those.

Like Bob Proctor says: "If you want to improve the quality of your life, start allocating a portion of each day to changing your paradigm."

- **IDENTIFY 'TROUBLESOME THOUGHTS'**

Identify the feelings that bring you problems, and seek to prevent and change them. Let them stop intentionally by saying 'no' out loud. It may sound silly, but that simple action breaks your chain of thought and helps you to introduce a new, safer one. The easiest way to do so is to count as many times as you like from one to 100 until your negative thoughts go away.

- **DON'T STEP ON THE SCALE**

Even though stepping on the scale to check on your progress is not bad, many people often associate it with negative thoughts. If you know the number on the scale will lead to negative and self-destructive thoughts, then you should avoid it. At least until you are in a place where the number on the scale doesn't affect your mental health.

- **FORGET ABOUT THE ENTIRE 'FOODS' ATTITUDE**

We've learned somewhere along the way to feel either proud or bad for any food choice we make. But in the end, it's just food, so you shouldn't feel bad for enjoying an occasional cookie. Permit yourself to have a piece of chocolate cake or a glass of wine sometimes.

Treating yourself to some comfort food is right for your mind and body. It is doing it every day that sabotages weight loss. During a more or less strict diet, having a day in a week to get away from is the key to success, the guarantee for motivation, and does not undermine the goal of losing weight.

- **FOCUS ON THE ATTAINABLE**

If you've never been to a gym before, your goal on day one shouldn't be to do 30 minutes on the elliptical. Going for a 30-minute walk might be a better goal. If you want to cook more but have little familiarity with healthier cooking, don't bank on creating new nutritious recipes every night after work. Instead, consider using a subscription service such as Blue Apron or HelloFresh, where pre-portioned recipes and ingredients are delivered to your doorstep, helping you get to know different components, make new meals, and develop your cooking skills.

- **ENVISION A BETTER LIFE**

What will life be like if you put good habits in place? Will you be more comfortable in your clothes? Will it give you more energy? Will you sleep better? Will you laugh more? Will you be happier? Will you be a better wife or mum? Attempt to get as thorough and realistic as possible. How will your life change if you changed your lifestyle?

Take a moment and sit down with a pen and ask yourself, what do I want? What do I really want? Write it down and make a written description of it in the present tense. Build a vision of what you would like to accomplish.

Take time to visualize a better life in the beginning and throughout your weight loss plan. Changing your habits is hard, so why bother if it doesn't bring you something new and better. Imagine a better life that will start giving you something to look forward to as well as work towards. See what you want, get a picture of it in your mind. Vision is going to direct your life.

- ## BELIEVE IN YOUR VISION

This is important. There's no point in having a vision unless you think it will come true. With almost everything, you have to believe that you can make this happen. So you can change your lifestyle, lose weight, and hope for a better future. To be successful, you have to believe you can do it without anybody else evaluation. You have to believe in what you see. Keep your vision up front, and think it's waiting for you. You have to persist and persevere in working on what you want to achieve. That'll keep you focused and move on.

Imagining a happier future makes you hopeful – although things go wrong sometimes, you will just have to hope it's for the greater good. Learning not to focus on the bad will help you stay focused on living a healthier lifestyle.

Sacrifice is giving up something of a lower nature, to receive something of a higher nature. Sacrifice is based on faith, and if you have faith, you will take action.

- ## BELIEVE YOU ARE IN CONTROL

You must realize you control your life. You have to take responsibility for your actions to excel in losing weight and other goals – you have to trust that you are in charge. If you put your future in other people's hands, you will never be able to move on. Of course, there are always circumstances out of our control, but your type of reaction is up to you.

While taking control of your life is empowering, it's also frightening because if you don't achieve your goal, you have no one to blame but yourself. "No one has control over your life – but you."

• GET TO LEARN HOW TO COPE

Many of your problems with weight loss are from your physio-logical reactions to stress. Most times, you crave spaghetti or candy when you have a bad day. Or you order a pizza becau-se there was nothing to cook for dinner. Or give up on losing weight when work gets busy, or when you get to some other stressful season of life.

When you want to lose weight, life doesn't just continue ef-fortlessly without stress. Sadly, life will never be secure, and there will always be a pain. Consequently, if you fall off track each time, life does not go your way, then it is time you learn new coping strategies. The goal is to maintain a healthy life-style and lose weight, no matter the obstacles life throws our way.

If the way you cope with stress keeps you from putting new behaviors in place or maintaining them, you might want to talk to a therapist or counselor. A therapist or psychologist will help you develop healthier coping skills and work through stress. This will help you free up space in your brain to focus on that better life. Having excellent optimistic coping skills is necessary for growth and surviving – not just for weight loss. Life is unpredictable and will not always go according to plan. Either you can get better or get bitter.

"The secret of success is learning how to use pain and pleasure instead of having pain and pleasure use you. If you do that, you're in control of your life. If you don't, life controls you." Tony Robbins

- **ELIMINATE THE CLUTTER AND THE CHAOS**

What do clutter and chaos have to do with weight loss? It's tough to picture a happier future when you are surrounded by confusion and noise. Clutter and confusion build hot zones, and when attempting to escape hot zones, it's challenging to develop new patterns and behaviors. Hot zones are moments when you feel stressed, overwhelmed, and the decisions you make are more about surviving the moment than on long-term goals.

- **CONCENTRATE ON SOLUTIONS AND NOT EXPLANA-TIONS**

A proactive approach that has been effective in the weight loss process is relying on options instead of excuses. You may be using excuses because you're scared of failing. So you say something like, "I can't get to the gym at that time" or "I 'm sick" or "That exercise never worked for me" instead of falling into an exercise routine. It offers you the freedom to either give up or not try at all. Failure, however, is part of the process. Failure is Good. And instead of making yourself give up, grant yourself the approval to lose. To succeed, you have to be okay with failure, not just at losing weight but in life in general.

HOW TO START IF? - STEP BY STEP GUIDE

Although intermittent fasting is a very simple and straightforward approach yet, fasting can be an intimidating word for many. Our dependence on food for our physical, mental, and emotional satisfaction has increased to such an extent that even the thought of abstinence from food can make people anxious. This is even more important in the case of women as controlling hunger for them can be very difficult. Their mind is internally programmed to look for food consciously.

This is a reason that although intermittent fasting is very easy and simple, some people may find it difficult to follow it in the long run.

The main reason some people may find intermittent fasting difficult to follow is not due to the severity of hunger or their inability to manage their routine but because they have not followed proper procedures.

Yes, you have read it right! The biggest reason people are unable to follow intermittent fasting is that they don't follow the process properly. They are so enthusiastic about losing weight that they don't give time to their bodies to prepare for the fasting schedules.

You must understand that humans have also evolved from animal species. Our first and foremost instinct is and always would be to eat, sleep, and procreate. If any obstruction is put in the way of either of these things, the initial reaction of our body would be adverse. If you try to snatch away any of these things or enforce stricter rules in these areas, the results are not going to be favorable.

No matter how beneficial fasting is for the body, the body is not going to react well to it initially. You will face hunger pangs, cramps, distraction, mind wandering around food, irritability, and mood swings. There are ways to manage all these symptoms, but there can be no denying the fact that these issues will arise.

You can lower these adverse reactions by following proper protocols, and intermittent fasting will become a life-changing experience for you. If you jump the steps and rush to the last part of the first leg, you are bound to have severe symptoms, and not only the results would get affected, but you will also face problems in managing the lifestyle for a long.

A STEP BY STEP APPROACH

The best way to approach intermittent fasting is to move step by step. You must never undermine the fact that our lifesty-les are heavily centered around food. There are shorter gaps between meals. There is a high amount of carb intake that also aggravates the situation to a great extent.

If you follow a very hard approach from the word GO, you are bound to face adjustment issues. The best approach is to allow the body to adapt to the fasting schedule and let it build the capacity to stay hungry.

- **ELIMINATE SNACKS**

This is something that would come several times in this book. It is a very important thing that you must understand. The root cause of most of our health issues is the habit of frequent snacking.

Snacking leads to 2 major issues:
1. It keeps causing repeated glucose spikes that invoke an in-sulin response and hence the overall insulin presence in the bloodstream increases aggravating the problem of insulin resistance.

2. It usually involves refined carb and sugar-rich food items that will lead to cravings and you will keep feeling the urge to eat at even shorter intervals.

This is a reason your preparation for intermittent fasting must begin with the elimination of snacks. You can have 2-3 nutrient-dense meals in a day, but you will have to remove the habit of snacking from your routine.

As long as the habit of snacking is there, you'll have a very hard time staying away from food as this habit never allows your ghrelin response clock to get set at fixed intervals. This means that you will keep having urges to eat sweets and car-b-rich foods, and you will also have strong hunger pangs at regular intervals.

The solution to this problem is very simple. You can take 2-3 nutrient-dense meals that are rich in fat, protein, and fiber. Such a meal will not only provide you with adequate energy for the day but would also keep your gut engaged for long so that you don't have frequent hunger pangs.

The farther you can stay away from refined carb-rich and su-gar-rich food items, the easier you would find it to deal with hunger.

You must start easy. Don't do anything drastic or earth-shat-tering.

Simply start by lowering the number of snacks you have in a day. The snacks have not only become a need of the body, but they are also a part of the habit. In a day, there are numerous instances when we eat tit-bits that we don't care about. We sip cold drinks, sweetened beverages, chips, cookies, bagels, donuts, burgers, pizzas simply because they are in front of us or accessible. We have made food an excuse to take breaks. This habit will have to be broken if you want to move on the path of good health.

- **WIDEN THE GAP BETWEEN YOUR MEALS**

This is the second step in your preparation. You must start widening the gap between your meals. This process needs to be gradual and should only begin when you have eliminated snacks from your routine. Two nutrient-dense meals in a day or two meals and a smaller meal or lunch comprising of fiber-rich salad should be your goal.

However, you must remember that these two steps must be ta-ken over a long period. You must allow your body to get used to the change. There would be a temptation that it is easy to follow these, and you can jump to the actual intermittent fa-sting routine, but it is very important to avoid all such temp-tations as they are only going to lead to failures.

If your body doesn't get used to this routine, very soon, you'll start feeling trapped. You'll start finding ways to cheat the routine. You'll look for excuses to violate the routine, and it very soon becomes a habit. This is the reason you must allow your body to take some time to adjust to the new schedule.

You should remember that intermittent fasting is a way of life. This might slower the results, but it is going to make your overall journey smoother and better.

THE BEST TIPS AND TRICKS FOR STARTING INTERMITTENT FASTING:

FOOD RELATED ASPECTS

- **Ensure You Are Fasting in a Healthy Way**

When it comes to fasting, it is important to ensure that you approach it in a way that will be beneficial for your health, and that will not do more harm than good. Firstly, you want to maintain flexibility with yourself and your body when fa-sting. If you are not feeling well as you are trying to fast, don't be afraid to eat a small amount on your fast days. This is espe-cially true at the beginning when you first introduce fasting into your diet.

- Increase Your Water Intake

You will also want to ensure you drink enough water each time you fast afterward. The recommendation is about two liters per day, but of course, this depends on your body size. In general, eight glasses of water that are about eight ounces each should give you enough water to be hydrated, but when fasting, this must increase to about nine to thirteen glasses. This works out to be between two or three liters of water.

- Avoid Eating Anything You Want After a Fast

Healthy meals should be your focus. They will help you get the required nutrients like vitamins, which will give you more energy during the fasting period. If you feel like you need to binge on unhealthy foods or large quantities after finishing a fast, it is time to reconsider your eating windows.

- Eat Only When Needed

When you can recognize when you eat without beginning hun-gry, you begin to create a discipline that you eat only when needed. The easiest way to do this is to build a schedule and then stick to it. Building a rather strict schedule will help your body remember to eat only when it is really needed. This ap-proach will go a long way in helping your stretch your fasting periods.

- Select the Foods You Eat Wisely

When you do break your fast or when you are eating small amounts on fasting days, choose the foods you eat wisely. You want to properly prepare your body to fast and keep it heal-thy while you do so. In addition to eating enough protein, you want to make sure that the other foods you eat are real, whole foods.

- Consider Supplementation

Supplementing may be very beneficial and even necessary when fasting to maintain and improve health. Some essential nutrients and minerals that your body would greatly benefit from, like Omega-3's or iron, may be challenging to get in ade-quate amounts if you are fasting. For this reason, supplemen-ting them may benefit you in terms of keeping you feeling he-althy and energetic, as well as keeping your brain functioning to its full potential.

- Start Small

If you have never tried it before, there is no way you can start fasting and go for a whole 48 hours without a meal. You can start with a 10- or 12-hour window first, having your food at 8 pm, for example, and having nothing again until 8 am the next day. It will be easier since sleep is incorporated into your eating window.

PERSONAL ASPECTS

- Pay Attention to Your Body

If you feel unwell while you are fasting, it is important to stop and check what could be the issue. It is normal to feel tired, hungry, and maybe irritable when you fast, but you may want to stop your fast if you feel unwell or weak. To be safe, for your first few times fasting, keep the duration shorter, and work your way up to the desired amount of time.

- Keep Yourself Busy

During the fasting period, try to find something that will keep you busy as it will help take your mind off food. Go for long walks, catch up with friends, do gardening, stay busy at work or pick up new hobbies.

- Patience

You need to be patient with your intermittent fasting journey, and it will take a few days or weeks to feel like the "new nor-mal". Try to be consistent with your meal calendar, and it will get simpler.

- Ensure You Get Enough Sleep

When you get enough sleep, you can be healthier, and your overall well-being is guaranteed. When we sleep, the body runs certain functions in the body that help burn calories and improve the metabolic rate. Make sure you get your recom-mended hours of sleep every night.

- Holistic Support

Holistic support is a topic that is particularly dear to me. Here I will offer you, because of limited space, just a few hints, but I invite you, if you are interested, in exploring these issues.

As I have already told you, I am convinced that there are many ways which guide us towards our goals. Nutrition and the practice of intermittent fasting are very important, but they are not the only ones. We must aim at attaining complete spiritual harmony as well as physical well-being

- Yoga

Yoga is a useful therapeutic tool to know and understand what is happening, to become observers of one's changing body, and to enter into harmony with ourselves and our needs. The practice can represent a rebirth especially for those who have never approached yoga. The advantages that the constant practice of yoga can provi-de are very powerful:

- relieves pain resulting from typical age-related illness, such as osteoporosis and arthritis
- meditative practice and slow breathing allow you to reach a state of serenity that involves a natural lowering of blood pressure
- relief of chronic back pain
- fights depression
- reduces the time it takes to fall asleep

Here are the most recommended asanas (body posture) for menopausal yoga:

- **Baddha Konasana** (position of the butterfly) indicated for meditation, easy to hold, and ideal for breathing. It works on the kidneys and bladder and tones the muscles that support the internal organs. Perfect position to reduce the discomforts of menopause.

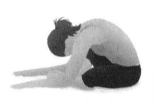

- **Dandasana** (posture of the stick). Another gentle position.Effective to prevent digestive problems and those related to sciatica.

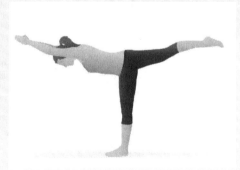

- **Trikonasana** (position of the triangle). This position involves a torsion of the torso and is contraindicated in the case of minor disorders of the spine and knees. One of its benefits is the reduction of blood pressure; it also tones the arms and legs muscles.

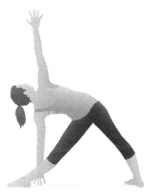

- **Tadasana** (position of the mountain). It is one of the basic positions of yoga: it is safe and does not involve twisting. It relaxes all the back muscles, helps develop balance, and works the abdominal muscles, promoting digestion and improving posture. We advise you not to keep your arms raised for too long, especially if you have suffered any shoulder injuries.

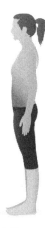

MEDITATION

The goal of meditation is to reach a level of greater aware-ness and inner calm. You learn to be able to focus attention on yourself, following perceptions, sensations, thoughts, and emo-tions, or on the external environment. Meditation is just that: focusing on the here and now, without unnecessary anxieties, worries and thoughts. Meditating means enjoying the present moment and disciplining the mind to detach itself from its "autopilot" to contemplate what surrounds us and feel all the sensations that pass Meditation is a great way to stay motivated. It is a healthy way to build positive energy inside you and chase away the negative thoughts. Practicing meditation for a few minutes daily can help you focus on achieving your goals

ESSENTIAL OILS

Essential oils have been found to be an important means of improving mental health. Many studies show their effective-ness. Combined with consistent self-care, essential oils can en-rich our lives and improve the state of our overall well-being. The aroma of essential oils can bring back vivid memories of the past as well as create visceral responses in the body that promote healing. Research conducted in 2007 found that one massage per week with essential oils, performed on the abdo-men, arms, and back, offers the first benefits for the symp-toms of menopause after about 8 sessions. Alternatively, you can put 2 or 3 drops a day or every other day on the sole of the foot or on the pulse points.

Another option is to dilute 2 or 3 drops with water and put them in a diffuser, so that their essence is diffused in the air.

Below you will find some of the benefits they can bring:

- Pine essential oil: Research published in April 2003 in The Bone Journal showed that this oil reduces bone fragility, managing to prevent osteoporosis.

- Lavender essential oil: promotes relaxation and sleep. It reduces the anxiety induced by menopause by relieving hot flashes, headaches, and palpitations.

- Rose essential oil improves mood and reduces hot flashes by balancing hormones.

- Geranium essential oil: promotes hormonal balance and regularity of the menstrual cycle in perimenopause. It is also effective on mood.

MUSIC THERAPY

The beauty and depth of human expression through art and music can be moving and awe-inspiring. Listen to singers whose voices you find truly unique and beautiful. Put on an opera or a symphony with a fabulous, sweeping fifinale. Look at paintings and sculptures that are stunning in their aesthetic, technique, or capture of emotion. Read poetry that touches you with its sincerity and creativity. If no artists or artworks come to mind right away, that's perfectly OK. Think of art and music as a therapeutic path to explore, with the goal of discovering a few creations that inspire a transformative sense of awe.

Sound, like energy, has the ability to resonate with the energy of surrounding bodies. When the vibration emitted is in resonance with the vibration of the receiver, then harmony is generated.

We as human beings are energetic beings, therefore we emit vibrations as each of our organs vibrate at their own frequency. If a person is in a disharmonious state and resonates with a harmonic frequency, he/she will gradually normalize back to the original frequency.

For this reason, when we listen to sounds at 432 Hz, we resonate with this frequency creating a harmonious and balancing effect for our organism.

In fact, music at 432 Hz can also be used for therapeutic purposes. Being harmonically tuned in with the biophysical processes of the organism, we are promoting the healing process.

EXERCISING

Exercise can be done when fasting, but it is not a must. Mild exercises can be done even at home. By exercising, you will build your muscle strength, and your body fat will burn faster.

Physical activity counteracts the loss of bone mass and increases its density. Thus helping to prevent osteoporosis. It also strengthens muscle tone and improves balance and posture, allowing for safer movements. Regular physical activity, even if moderate, also promotes mental health as it increases the levels of ß-endorphins, neurotransmitters that raise the mood and reduce hot flashes and sweating. In the next chapter, you will find a series of exercises that can support and reinforce the benefits of intermittent fasting.

MOTIVATIONAL ASPECTS

Your Mindset

The first and probably the biggest tip I can give you for intermittent fasting is to go into it with a positive mindset.

But what is the mindset?

The Mindset is a mental inclination, a way of thinking that affects the mood, the way of acting. This will guide your choices and the results you will achieve. Your mind collects ideas, thoughts, and beliefs. These define your personality and your behavior. Your mind has a very strong power because it makes you see things not in an objective way, but as you perceive them. First of all, we need to establish clearly and in detail what the goals we want to achieve are and why we want to do so. Once we understand this aspect, the right mindset is needed to give us energy and put us in a position to find all the necessary tools to achieve our goal. Our mindset massively affects the way we face life and the challenges we go through, affecting our success or failure. So if at this moment you are reading this book understanding the enormous benefits that intermittent fasting can bring to your life, but you are convinced that you cannot do it, or that nothing can change the situation you are in, or you are convinced that this will only work for other women but not for you, you most likely won't make it. I'm not saying this because I can predict the future, but simply because I know that our thoughts shape our behaviors. Perhaps Gandhi's words could make you think: "Your mind is everything, what you think you become". Therefore it is important that you understand that you are creating your change, and you are deciding your success.

Let me briefly explain how you might start changing your mindset. To be able to reach our goals it is imperative to establish an effective daily routine:

• Clearly identify the goal you want to achieve. Write it down and observe it for a few minutes a day, it will serve to motivate and energize you.

- Visualize the goal you want to achieve and how this will change your life. How do you feel? Is it worth fighting foryour goal? As you will understand, no one achieves its go-als overnight. So once you know what you're aiming for, set a plan of smaller, more easily achievable goals.

- Set and write down daily, weekly, and monthly goals on a calendar. The goals, especially the daily and weekly ones, must be realistic and achievable, otherwise, failing to reach them, will result in discouragement and will require a grea-ter effort to stay on track.

- Strive every day to take actions that bring us closer to our goal.

- Establish a daily priority list, this will help you not to wa-ste your energy on activities that are not useful in achie-ving your purpose.

- Collect any information that may be useful to you.

- Remember that every result achieved requires effort, nothing happens if we do not work for it.

- Always keep in mind that no excuses are accepted: there is nothing we cannot do; we are able, just like any other people, to improve and achieve our personal goals; we are not less fortunate than others; we deserve to be happy just like all other people.

So, let's get to work!!!

PROFESSIONAL ADVICE

If you require medicine in the morning that needs food, some intermittent fasting protocols might not be for you. If you have any other serious health conditions that restrict your eating habits, then you should talk to your doctor first.

KEEP TRACK OF YOUR ACHIEVEMENTS

Keep track of your achievements by using a regular notebook. There is something about writing things down on paper that makes it highly personal.

When you do this, you can see how you have been progressing. Make sure to write down the date and the length of each fast.

Also, include some notes about the things that went right and the things that didn't go right. That way, you can see how your intermittent fasting regimen has been affecting you both positively and negatively.

SELF-REWARD WHEN REACHING SMALL TARGETS

Set yourself up for progress by utilizing a prize framework. For example:

- After shedding fifteen pounds, get yourself some new clothes.

- If you meet all your monthly goals, treat yourself to a massage.

The cash spared by skipping a meal (or two) can pay for your prize! The things that can motivate us are different for every one of us, so make sure to pick something that works best for you, and you will stay focused on reaching all of your goals.

WHAT TO EAT AFTER FASTING

Eating after you've fasted for a considerable amount of time can be challenging in a few ways. Not only do you have to ensure that you're eating nutrient-dense food but you must also be cautious of putting too much too soon on your digestive system.

This is why I'm including a list of foods that you can refer to when the time comes to eat something finally:

- **Healthy fats**: breaking your fast with healthy fats such as coconut and olive oil, avocados, eggs, ghee, and grass-fed butter will ensure that your digestive system is not overwhelmed and that you get the right nutrients that your body craves for after a fast.

- **Soups**: soups and broths aren't only good when you're fasting but can also be a great source of nutrients and vitamins when you're finally ready to eat again. While a simple veggie or bone broth can be your best friend during fasting, you can add a bunch of stuff like lentils, tofu or pasta to spice it up for the post-fasting period.

- **Veggies:** most of us don't need another long and boring lesson on the importance of consuming vegetables, but here it is again (I promise to keep it short though!). While all veggies are good for health, some starchy ones such as sweet potatoes can be a great source of resistant starches when breaking a fast. Just make sure that you cook them up thoroughly.

- **Smoothies:** These are a great way to give your body the nutrient punch it needs after fasting for several hours. What's more, smoothies are always fun to make since you can throw together almost anything and stir up a nutritious yet delicious drink in minutes. Not a vegetable person? Add in some romaine lettuce or spinach in your blend in order to prevent missing out on the benefits of these leafy greens without having to consume a bowl full of baked veggies instead.

- **Fermented foods**: foods such as unsweetened yogurt and kefir are a great source of probiotics that your gut is going to thank you over a million times for. Yogurt also contains almost all the nutrients that our bodies need, including but not limited to, calcium, B vitamins, proteins, phosphorus, and vitamin D. It is a precious source of trace minerals and is found to be particularly beneficial for osteoporosis and digestive health.

- **Fruits (fresh & dried):** to keep it light on your gut, you can also break your fast with fruits such as watermelon, grapes, and honeydew. These are ideal because they contain a high water content to combat dehydration and are easily digestible. If you want some inspiration from folks in other parts of the world then don't look beyond the Middle East and Arabia. People inhabiting these regions prefer to break their fasts with dates which are a dense source of nutrients and restore energy levels after a long fast. If dates are not your thing, try dried apricots or raisins for similar effects.

The above guide can be extremely helpful when one finally finds themselves in the eating window because it is pretty easy to get carried away by all those hunger pangs and eat whatever comes your way. However, I can guarantee from personal experience that if you let yourself indulge at that point, then you're going to regret it later.

It only takes a few minutes of mindless eating to come back to your senses and realize that you've just spoiled everything you worked for till that point.

Meal planning is very important for this reason; when you don't know what kind of healthy meal awaits you at the end of your fast, you're more prone to eating whatever comes your way regardless of the consequences.

The end result may look something like this:

Snacking --- Guilt ---Eating --- More Guilt (and the cycle continues on to more snacking)

You definitely do not want that!

CHAPTER 5

INTERMITTENT FASTING AND EXERCISE

Yet many may wonder if it's safe to exercise during an intermittent fast. With the body depleted of nutrients during a fast after all, would it be wise to put it through any more strain than it is already under? According to the data, exercise while undergoing a fast has a direct effect on metabolism and the body's level of insulin. Both are activated with one going up and the other going down as the body re-calibrates and begins to burn fat rather than carbs. Engaging in the right kind of workout will help to speed up this process even more. Having that said, here are some exercises to give your intermittent fast a major boost.

RUNNING/TREADMILL

There is really nothing better to get the body's metabolic cylinders running than a good run. As soon as your feet hit the pavement (or the treadmill), your heart rate increases and the blood starts to much more vigorously pump through your body. With your bodily processes instantly speeding up like this, it's no wonder that your metabolism might speed up as well. And this is precisely the case when you engage in this type of exercise during a fast. But having that said, just keep in mind that you have to be careful not to overdo it. And in order to ensure that you have the best experience, it of your fast. That way, your body still has plenty of additio-nal resources left over from the last meal you had before your fast began. If for example, you begin your fast at 10 PM on a Thursday night, you should be good to run around the block at 7 AM Friday morning without any trouble. It is not advisable, however, to overexert yourself at the very end of your fast. Although most could probably handle it, to be on the safe few hours of your fast every step you take causes hormones to alert your metabolic engines that you are up and entirely running.

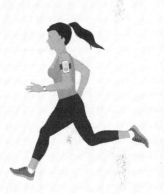

WEIGHTLIFTING

If you are a weightlifter or interested in becoming one, have some good news. Lifting weights does not interfere with your fast! Lifting weights during a fast can prove quite benefits. Intermittent fasting is designed to prevent muscle loss during fasting periods. Still, having that said, a little weightlifting will help to shield your body from muscle loss even more. Because the truth is, we all lose muscle as we age. If we don't work at maintaining it through muscle lifting, we just might lifting weights during an intermittent fast also quickens the pace of fat burn even more.

Just think about it, during a fast your body has already switched to burning fat for its fuel, so when you grunt, struggle, and strain to lift those weights, guess what your body's tapping into for energy? All that fat you want to get rid of!

PUSH-UP

One of the most traditional exercises you could ever even consider would be that of the classic pushup. Push-ups have been around forever and there is a reason for that they are highly effective. By making use of gravity and your own body weight, the push-up gets the heart going while the muscles arm strength alone. These exercises if done moderately say no more than 20 to 30 pushups during a fast can be highly effective in boosting your metabolism to the max, allowing an even more rapid depletion of the body's fat stores. This is some good news that you could most certainly use!

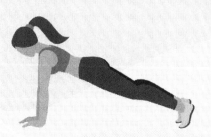

SQUATS

This is another great exercise that seems absolutely made for intermittent fasting. Squats focus on your glutes, quads, and other muscles like there is no tomorrow! This exercise keeps you going and keeps you strong! As you might imagine, squats consist of the participant bending their knees and squatting down toward the ground as if they are sitting on a chair. This bending motion gets the blood flowing to the thighs and be-gins rapidly burning fat deposits. If you need to target fat in the legs, in particular, you might want to give this exercise a try.

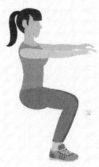

DIPS

Why yes we would be remiss if we did not mention dips! And no, I'm not talking about the stuff you dip your chips in at the football game, I'm talking about high-intensity, fat busing exercise that will burn fat, boost your metabolism, and make sure your upper body stays nice and strong. These exercises are just about perfect for intermittent fasting as they get.

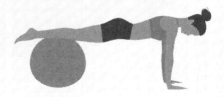

PLANKS

Planks can be done at home, at the gym, or just about any place you may be at the time. This exercise is also quite nuanced and of focus. Planks tend to build up quite a bit of endurance too, which is most certainly good for someone who is undergoing hours of your fast, but they can be done periodically throughout the rest of the fasting day as well.

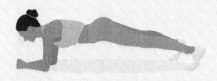

REVERSE LUNGE

Reverse lunges are a high-intensity workout that gets your metabolism going. And when done during a fast, it really kicks things into high gear. They are also good for getting your legs aerobic exercise you could do.

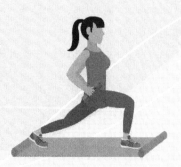

BURPEE

The Burpee is a classic hybrid-styled exercise that makes full use of cardio as well as resistance exercises, in order to maximize your metabolism. These exercises are pret-ty intensive, so if you are engaged in a less than 500 calorie fast day, you might want actually to have a low-calorie snack or other healthy option. Good choices for nutrition before this workout would be perhaps just a 1 hard-boiled egg, a salad, or maybe even a bowl of chicken broth. Either way, these wor-kouts are sure to get your body running on all cylinders during your intermittent fast.

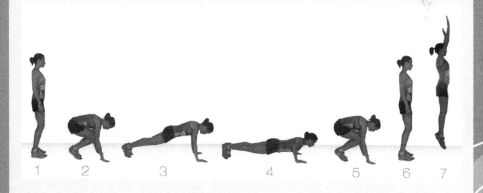

1   2   3   4   5   6   7

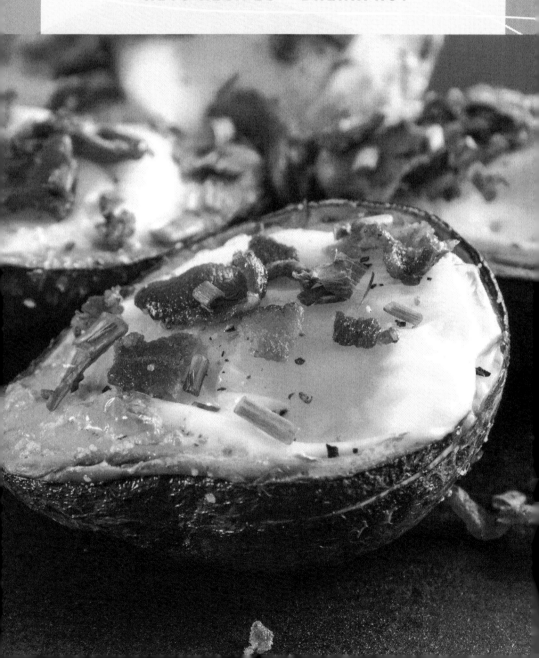

CHAPTER 6

KETO RECIPES - BREAKFAST

SAUSAGE OMELET

PREPARATION TIME: 15 MIN   **COOKING TIME: 20 MIN**

SERVINGS: 4

INGREDIENTS

- ½ oz. gluten-free sausage links
- ½ cup heavy whipping cream
- Salt
- black pepper
- 8 large organic eggs
- 1 cup cheddar cheese
- 1/4 tsp. red pepper flakes

DIRECTIONS

1. Heat the oven to 350° F. Grease a baking dish. Cook the sausage for 8–10 minutes.
2. Put the rest of the ingredients in a bowl and beat. Remove sausage from the heat. Place cooked sausage in the baking dish then top with the egg mixture. Bake for 30 minutes. Slice and serve.

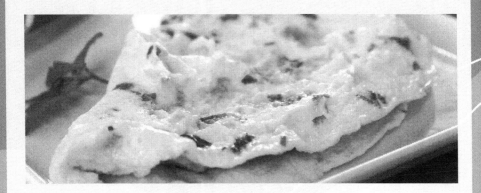

NUTRITION

- Calories: 334
- Carbs: 1.1g
- Protein: 20.6g

- Fat: 27.3g

BROWN HASH WITH ZUCCHINI

PREPARATION TIME: **10 MIN**   COOKING TIME: **20 MIN**

SERVINGS: **2**

INGREDIENTS

- 1 small onion
- 6 to 8 mushrooms
- 2 cups grass-fed ground beef
- 1 pinch of salt
- 1 pinch ground black pepper
- ½ tsp. smoked paprika
- 2 eggs

- 1 avocado
- 10 black olives
- 2 zucchini cut half

DIRECTIONS

1. Heat air fryer for 350° F. Grease a pan with coconut oil. Add the onions, mushrooms, salt plus pepper to the pan. Add the ground beef and the smoked paprika and eggs.
2. Mix, then place the pan in Air Fryer. Set to cook for 18 to 20 minutes with a temperature, 375° F. Serve with chopped parsley and diced avocado!

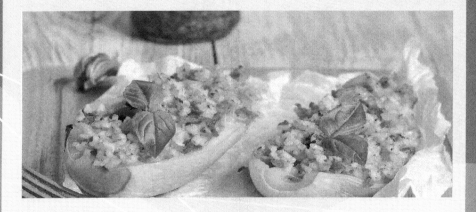

NUTRITION

- Calories: 290
- Carbs: 15g
- Protein: 20g

- Fat: 23g

CARROT BREAKFAST SALAD

PREPARATION TIME: 5 MIN   **COOKING TIME: 4 HOURS**

SERVINGS: 4

INGREDIENTS

- 2 tbsp. olive oil
- 2 oz. baby carrots, peeled and halved
- 3 garlic cloves, minced
- 2 yellow onions, chopped
- ½ cup vegetable stock
- 1/3 cup tomatoes, crushed
- A pinch of salt and black pepper

DIRECTIONS

1. In your slow cooker, combine all the ingredients, cover, and cook on high for 4 hours.
2. Divide into bowls and serve for breakfast.

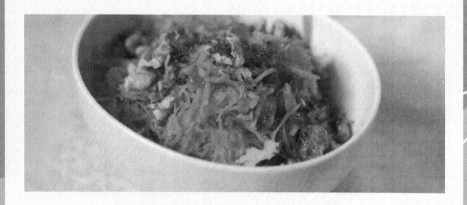

NUTRITION

- Calories: 437
- Protein: 2.39g
- Fat: 39.14g

- Carbs: 23.28g

DELICIOUS TURKEY WRAP

PREPARATION TIME: 10 MIN   COOKING TIME: 10 MIN

SERVINGS: 6

INGREDIENTS

- 1 ¼ oz. of ground turkey, lean
- 4 green onions, minced
- 1 tbsp. of olive oil
- 1 garlic clove, minced
- 2 tsp. of chili paste
- 8 oz. water chestnut, diced
- 3 tbsp. of hoisin sauce

- 2 tbsp. of coconut amino
- 1 tbsp. of rice vinegar
- 12 butter lettuce leaves
- 1/8 tsp. of salt

DIRECTIONS

1. Take a pan and place it over medium heat, add turkey and garlic to the pan
2. Heat for 6 minutes until cooked
3. Take a bowl and transfer turkey to the bowl
4. Add onions and water chestnuts
5. Stir in hoisin sauce, coconut amino, vinegar, and chili paste
6. Toss well and transfer the mix to lettuce leaves. Serve and enjoy.

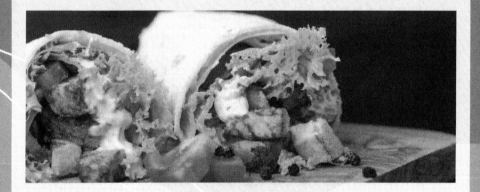

NUTRITION

- Calories: 162
- Fat: 4g
- Carbohydrates: 7g

- Protein: 23g

PUMPKIN PANCAKES

PREPARATION TIME: 10 MIN   **COOKING TIME: 15 MIN**

SERVINGS: 6

INGREDIENTS

- 3 Large eggs- Separate the egg whites for use
- 2/3 cups of organic oats
- 6 oz. pumpkin puree
- 1 scoop of collagen peptides
- 1 tsp. stevia powder
- ½ tsp. cinnamon
- Cooking spray

DIRECTIONS

1. Blend all the ingredients together to a smooth mixture.
2. Apply the cooking spray to the pan to coat it properly.
3. Pour a part of the batter into the pan and let it coat the pan properly
4. Wait till the edges of the pancake brown up a little bit
5. Flip it over and cook from the other side
6. You can serve it with fruits.

NUTRITION

- Calories: 70
- Carbs: 16g
- Fat: 3g

- Protein: 3g

LUNCH

BROCCOLI AND TURKEY DISH

PREPARATION TIME: 5 MIN　　　　　**COOKING TIME: 15 MIN**

SERVINGS: 2

INGREDIENTS

- 1/4 tsp. red pepper flakes
- 1 tbsp. olive oil
- 1 tsp. soy sauce
- 4 oz. broccoli florets
- 4 oz. cauliflower florets, riced
- 4 oz. ground turkey

DIRECTIONS

1. Bring out a skillet pan, place it over medium heat, add olive oil and when hot, add beef, crumble it and cook for 8 minutes until no longer pink.
2. Then add broccoli florets and riced cauliflower, stir well, drizzle with soy sauce and sesame oil, season with salt, black pepper, and red pepper flakes and continue cooking for 5 minutes until vegetables have thoroughly cooked.

NUTRITION

- Calories; 120.3
- Fat; 8.3g
- Protein: 8.4g
- Net Carb: 2g
- Fiber: 1g

EASY MAYO SALMON

PREPARATION TIME: 5 MIN   **COOKING TIME: 10 MIN**

SERVINGS: 2

INGREDIENTS

- 2 salmon fillets
- 4 tbsp. mayonnaise

DIRECTIONS

1. Turn on the Panini press, spray it with oil and let it preheat.
2. Then spread 1 tablespoon of mayonnaise on each side of salmon, place them on Panini press pan, shut with lid, and cook for 7 to 10 minutes until salmon has cooked to the desired level.

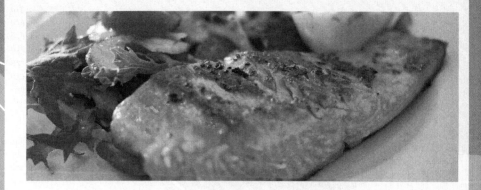

NUTRITION

- Cal 132.7
- Fats 11.1g
- Protein 8g
- Net Carb 0.3g

KETO BUFFALO CHICKEN EMPANADAS

PREPARATION TIME: 20 MIN   **COOKING TIME: 30 MIN**

SERVINGS: 6

INGREDIENTS

FOR THE EMPANADA DOUGH:
- 1 ½ cups mozzarella cheese
- 3 oz. cream cheese
- 1 whisked egg
- 2 cups almond flour

FOR THE BUFFALO CHICKEN FILLING:
- 2 cups shredded chicken
- 2 tbsp. Butter
- 0.33 cup Hot Sauce

DIRECTIONS

1. Heat the oven, 425° F. Microwave the cheese & cream cheese for 1-minute. Stir the flour and egg into the dish.
2. With another bowl, combine the chicken with sauce and set aside.
3. Cover a flat surface with plastic wrap and sprinkle with almond flour.
4. Grease a rolling pin, press the dough flat. Make the circle shapes out of this dough with a lid. Portion out spoonfuls of filling into these dough circles.
5. Fold the other half over to close up into half-moon shapes.
6. Bake for 9 minutes. Serve.

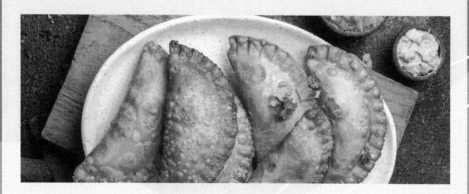

NUTRITION

- Net carbs: 20g
- Fiber: 0g
- Fat: 96g
- Protein: 74g
- Calories: 1217

PEPPERONI AND CHEDDAR STROMBOLI

PREPARATION TIME: 15 MIN   **COOKING TIME: 20 MIN**

SERVINGS: 3

INGREDIENTS

- 1.25 cups Mozzarella Cheese
- 0.25 cup Almond Flour
- 3 tbsp. Coconut Flour
- 1 tsp. Italian Seasoning
- 1 Egg
- 6 oz. Deli Ham
- 2 oz. Pepperoni

- 4 oz. Cheddar Cheese
- 1 tbsp. Butter
- 6 cups Salad Greens

DIRECTIONS

1. Heat the oven, 400° F.
2. Melt the mozzarella. Mix flours and Italian seasoning in a separate bowl.
3. Dump in the melty cheese and mix with pepper and salt.
4. Stir in the egg and process the dough. Pour it onto that prepared baking tray.
5. Roll out the dough. Cut slits that mark out 4 equal rectangles.
6. Put the ham and cheese, then brush with butter and close up.
7. Bake for 17 minutes. Slice and serve.

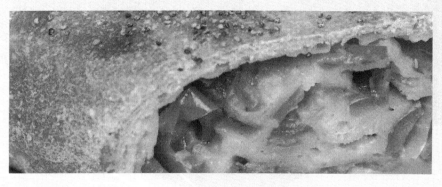

NUTRITION

- Net carbs: 20g
- Fiber: 0g
- Fat: 13g

- Protein: 11g
- Calories: 240

ZESTY AVOCADO AND LETTUCE SALAD

PREPARATION TIME: 5 MIN   **COOKING TIME: 0 MIN**

SERVINGS: 2

INGREDIENTS

- ½ of a lime, juiced
- 1 avocado, pitted, sliced
- 2 tbsp. olive oil
- 4 oz. chopped lettuce
- 4 tbsp. chopped chives

DIRECTIONS

1. Prepare the dressing and for this, bring out a small bowl, add oil, lime juice, salt, and black pepper, stir until mixed, and then slowly mix oil until combined.
2. Bring out a large bowl, add avocado, lettuce, and chives, and then toss gently.
3. Drizzle with dressing, toss until well coated and then serve.

NUTRITION

- Calories: 125.7
- Fat: 11g
- Protein: 1.3g
- Net Carb: 1.7g
- Fiber: 3.7g

DINNER

CILANTRO LIME FLOUNDER

PREPARATION TIME: 20 MIN   **COOKING TIME: 6 MIN**

SERVINGS: 3

INGREDIENTS

- ¼ cup homemade mayonnaise (here)
- 1 lime juice Zest
- 1½ cup fresh cilantro
- 3 (3-oz.) flounder fillets

DIRECTIONS

1. Preheat the oven to 300°F. Stir the mayonnaise, lime juice, lime zest, and cilantro in a small bowl.
2. Place 3 pieces of foil on a clean work surface, about 8 by 8 inches square. In the center of each square, place a flounder fillet.
3. Top the fillets with the mixture of mayonnaise evenly. Season the pepper to the flounder. Fold the foil sides over the fish, create a snug packet, and place on a baking sheet the foil packets.
4. Bake the fish for three to six minutes. Unfold and display the boxes.

NUTRITION

- Fat: 3g
- Carbohydrates: 2g;
- Phosphorus: 208g
- Potassium: 138g
- Sodium: 268g
- Protein: 12g

SEAFOOD CASSEROLE

PREPARATION TIME: **20 MIN**   COOKING TIME: **36 MIN**

SERVINGS: **6**

INGREDIENTS

- 2 cups sliced eggplant
- Cut 1 inch bits of butter
- 1 tbsp. of olive oil
- ½ small sweet onion
- 1 tbsp. of minced garlic
- 1 celery stalk
- ½ red bell pepper
- 3 tbsp. of freshly squeezed lemon

- juice
- 1 tbsp. of hot sauce
- ¼ tbsp. of Creole Seasoning Mix (here)
- ½ cup of white rice,
- 1 large egg
- 3 oz. of cooked shrimp.

DIRECTIONS

1. Cook the eggplant for 6 minutes in a small saucepan filled with water over medium-high heat. Drain in a large bowl and set aside.
2. Grease and set aside an 8-by-13-inch butter baking dish. Heat the olive oil in a large pot over medium heat.
3. Drizzle the onion, garlic, celery, and pepper bell for about 3 minutes or until tender. In addition to the lemon juice, hot sauce, Creole seasoning, rice, and egg, add the sautéed vegetables to the eggplant.
4. Remove to combine. Fold in the meat of the crab and shrimp.
5. In the casserole dish, spoon the casserole mixture and pat down the top. Bake for 26 to 40 minutes until the casserole is heated through and the rice is tender. Serve hot.

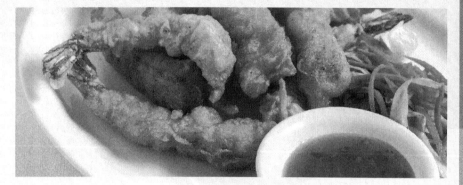

NUTRITION

- Fat: 3g
- Carbohydrates: 8g
- Phosphorus: 102g

- Potassium: 188g
- Sodium: 236g
- Protein: 12g

HERB PESTO TUNA

PREPARATION TIME: **10 MIN**   COOKING TIME: **10 MIN**

SERVINGS: **3**

INGREDIENTS

- 3 oz yellow fin tuna fillet z
- 1 tbsp. olive oil
- Freshly ground black pepper
- ¼ cup Herb Pesto (see here)
- 1 lemon, cut into 8 thin slices

DIRECTIONS

1. Heat to medium-high barbecue. Add the olive oil to the fish and season the fillet with pepper. On the barbecue, cook it for 3 minutes. Turn over the fish and top each piece using the herb slices. Grill until the tuna is cooked to medium-well for 6 to 6 minutes longer.
2. Modification of dialysis: The pesto adds to this recipes about 16 mg of potassium. The tuna is the reason why the potassium recipe is high. Try this recipe with other fish like haddock or cod, but instead of putting it on the barbecue, broil the fish. recipe with other fish lir cod, but instead of putting it on the barbecue, broil the fish.

NUTRITION

- Calories: 190
- Carbs: 7g
- Fat: 2g
- Phosphorus: 236g
- Sodium: 38g

GRILLED CALAMARI WITH LEMON AND HERBS

PREPARATION TIME: **10 MIN**   COOKING TIME: **3 MIN**

SERVINGS: **3**

INGREDIENTS

- 2 tbsp. of olive oil
- 2 tbsp. of freshly squeezed lemon juice
- 1 tbsp. of chopped fresh parsley
- 1 tbsp. of chopped fresh oregano
- 2 tbsp. of minced garlic

DIRECTIONS

1. Pinch sea salt Pinch freshly ground black pepper ½ pound of cleaned calamari Lemon wedges, to be garnished In a large bowl, combine olive oil, lemon juice, petroleum, oregano, garlic, salt, and pepper.
2. In the bowl, add the calamari and stir to coat. Cover the bowl and cool the calamari to marinate for 1 hour.
3. Preheat to medium-high the barbecue. Grill the calamari for about 3 minutes, turning once, until firm and opaque. Serve with wedges of lemon.

NUTRITION

- Fat: 8g
- Carbohydrates: 2g
- Phosphorus: 128g
- Potassium: 160g
- Sodium: 68g
- Protein: 3g

TRADITIONAL CHICKEN VEGETABLE SOUP

PREPARATION TIME: **20 MIN**   COOKING TIME: **36 MIN**

SERVINGS: **1**

INGREDIENTS

- 1 tbsp. of unsalted butter
- ½ sweet onion,
- 2 tbsp. of chopped garlic
- 2 celery stalks,
- 1 carrot chopped,
- 2 cups of chicken breast chopped
- 1 cup of Easy Chicken Stock

- (here)
- 3 cups of water
- 1 tbsp. of freshly chopped thyme
- Black pepper freshly ground
- 2 tbsp. of chopped fresh parsley

DIRECTIONS

1. Melt the butter in a large pot over medium heat. Sauté the onion and garlic for about 3 minutes until softened.
2. Add celery, carrot, chicken, stuffed chicken, and water. Bring the soup to a boil, reduce heat, and simmer until the vegetables are tender for about 40 minutes.
3. Add the thyme and cook the soup for 2 minutes. Season with pepper and serve with parsley on top.

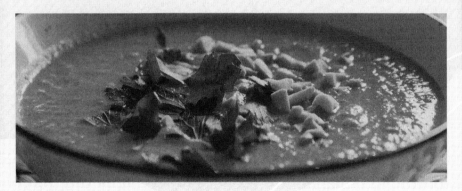

NUTRITION

- Fat: 6g
- Carbohydrates: 2g
- Phosphorus: 108g

- Potassium: 188g
- Sodium: 62g
- Protein: 16g

SNACK

KETO COCONUT FLAKE BALLS

PREPARATION TIME: 15 MIN   **COOKING TIME: 0 MIN**

SERVINGS: 2

INGREDIENTS

- 1 vanilla shortbread collagen protein bar
- 1 tbsp. lemon
- ¼ tsp. ground ginger
- ½ cup unsweetened coconut flakes
- ¼ tsp. ground turmeric

DIRECTIONS

1. Process protein bar, ginger, turmeric, and 3/4 of the total fflakes into a food processor.
2. Remove and add a spoon of water and roll till dough forms.
3. Roll into balls, and sprinkle the rest of the flakes on it. Serve.

NUTRITION

- Calories: 204
- Total Fat: 11g
- Total Carbs: 4.2g
- Protein: 1.5g

CREAMY SPINACH

INGREDIENTS

- 2 garlic cloves, peeled and minced
- 8 oz. of spinach leaves
- A drizzle of olive oil
- Salt and ground black pepper, to taste
- 4 tbsp. sour cream
- 1 tbsp. butter
- 2 tbsp. Parmesan cheese, grated

DIRECTIONS

1. Heat a pan with the oil over medium heat, add the spinach, stir and cook until it softens.
2. Add the salt, pepper, butter, Parmesan cheese, and butter, stir, and cook for 4 minutes.
3. Add the sour cream, stir, and cook for 5 minutes.
4. Divide between plates and serve.

NUTRITION

- Calories: 233
- Fat: 10g
- Fiber: 4g
- Carbohydrates: 4g
- Protein: 2g

AVOCADO FRIES

PREPARATION TIME: 10 MIN **COOKING TIME: 5 MIN**

SERVINGS: 3

INGREDIENTS

- 3 avocados, pitted, peeled, halved, and sliced
- 1½ cups sunflower oil
- 1½ cups almond meal
- A pinch of cayenne pepper
- Salt and ground black pepper, to taste

DIRECTIONS

1. In a bowl, mix the almond meal with salt, pepper, and cayenne, and stir. In a second bowl, whisk eggs with a pinch of salt and pepper.
2. Dredge the avocado pieces in egg and then in almond meal mixture. Heat a pan with the oil over medium-high heat, add the avocado fries, and cook them until they are golden.
3. Transfer to paper towels, drain grease, and divide between plates, and serve.

NUTRITION

- Calories: 200
- Fat: 43g
- Fiber: 4g
- Carbs: 7g
- Protein: 17g

BELL PEPPER NACHOS

PREPARATION TIME: 15 MIN   COOKING TIME: 10 MIN

SERVINGS: 2

INGREDIENTS

- 2 bell peppers
- 4 oz. beef ground
- ¼ tsp. cumin
- ¼ cup guacamole
- salt
- 1 cup cheese
- ¼ tsp. chili powder

- 1 tbsp. vegetable oil
- 2 tbsp. sour cream
- ¼ cup Pico de Gallo

DIRECTIONS

1. Put the bell peppers in a microwave dish, sprinkle salt and splash water on it and microwave for 4 minutes and cut it into 4 pieces.
2. Toast the chili powder and cumin in the pan for 30 seconds. Put the salted beef, stir and cook for 4 minutes. Put on all the pieces of pepper. Add cheese and cook for 1 minute. Serve with Pico de Gallo, guacamole, and cream.

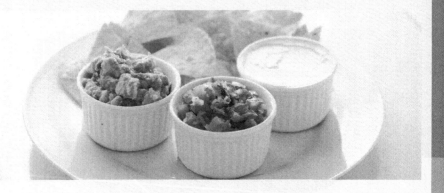

NUTRITION

- Calories: 475
- Carbs: 19g
- Fat: 24g

- Protein: 50g

CHAPTER 7
VEGETARIAN RECIPES - BREAKFAST

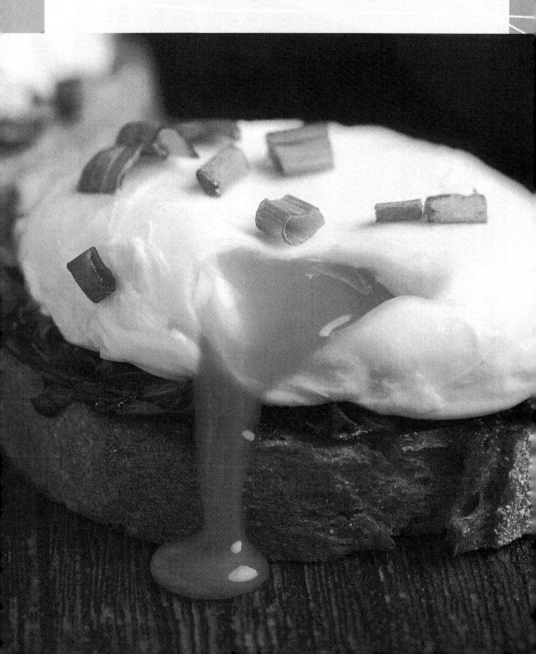

QUINOA BLACK BEANS BREAKFAST BOWL

PREPARATION TIME: 5-15 MIN   COOKING TIME: 25 MIN

SERVINGS: 4

INGREDIENTS

- 1 cup brown quinoa, rinsed well
- Salt to taste
- 3 tbsp. plant-based yogurt
- ½ lime, juiced
- 2 tbsp. chopped fresh cilantro
- 1 (5 oz.) can black beans, drained and rinsed
- 3 tbsp. tomato salsa
- ¼ small avocado, pitted, peeled, and sliced
- 2 radishes, shredded
- 1 tbsp. pepitas (pumpkin seeds)

DIRECTIONS

1. Cook the quinoa with 2 cups of slightly salted water in a medium pot over medium heat or until the liquid absorbs, 15 minutes.
2. Spoon the quinoa into serving bowls and fluff with a fork.
3. In a small bowl, mix the yogurt, lime juice, cilantro, and salt. Divide this mixture on the quinoa and top with beans, salsa, avocado, radishes, and pepitas.
4. Serve immediately.

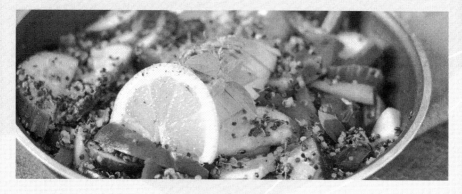

NUTRITION

- Calories: 131
- Fat; 3.5g
- Carbs: 20
- Protein: 6.5g

CORN GRIDDLECAKES WITH TOFU MAYONNAISE

PREPARATION TIME: 5-15 MIN   **COOKING TIME: 35 MIN**

SERVINGS: 4

INGREDIENTS

- 1 tbsp. flax seed powder + 3 tbsp. water
- 1 cup water or as needed
- 2 cups yellow cornmeal
- 1 tsp. salt
- 2 tsp. baking powder
- 4 tbsp. olive oil for frying
- 1 cup tofu mayonnaise for serving

DIRECTIONS

1. In a medium bowl, mix the flax seed powder with water and allow thickening for 5 minutes to form the flax egg.
2. Mix in the water and then whisk in the cornmeal, salt, and baking powder until the soup texture forms, but not watery.
3. Heat a quarter of the olive oil in a griddle pan and pour in a quarter of the batter. Cook until set and golden brown beneath, 3 minutes. Flip the cake and cook the other side until set and golden brown too.
4. Plate the cake and make three more with the remaining oil and batter.
5. Top the cakes with some tofu mayonnaise before serving.

NUTRITION

- Calories: 896
- Fat: 50. 7g
- Carbs: 91. 6g
- Protein: 17. 3g

LUNCH

KETO COCONUT FLAKE BALLS

INGREDIENTS

- 1 vanilla shortbread collagen protein bar
- 1 tbsp. lemon
- ¼ tsp. ground ginger
- ½ cup unsweetened coconut flakes,
- ¼ tsp. ground turmeric

DIRECTIONS

1. Process protein bar, ginger, turmeric, and ¾ of the total flakes into a food processor.
2. Remove and add a spoon of water and roll till dough forms.
3. Roll into balls, and sprinkle the rest of the flakes on it. Serve.

NUTRITION

- Calories: 204
- Total Fat: 11g
- Total Carbs: 4.2g

- Protein: 1.5g

CREAMY SPINACH

PREPARATION TIME: **10 MIN**   COOKING TIME: **15 MIN**

SERVINGS: **2**

INGREDIENTS

- 2 garlic cloves, peeled and minced
- 8 oz. of spinach leaves
- A drizzle of olive oil
- Salt and ground black pepper, to taste
- 4 tbsp. sour cream
- 1 tbsp. butter
- 2 tbsp. Parmesan cheese, grated

DIRECTIONS

1. Heat a pan with the oil over medium heat, add the spinach, stir and cook until it softens.
2. Add the salt, pepper, butter, Parmesan cheese, and butter, stir, and cook for 4 minutes.
3. Add the sour cream, stir, and cook for 5 minutes.
4. Divide between plates and serve.

NUTRITION

- Calories: 233
- Fat: 10g
- Fiber: 4g
- Carbohydrates: 4g
- Protein: 2g

TOMATO SAUCE WITH PUMPKIN

PREPARATION TIME: 10 MIN   **COOKING TIME: 15 MIN**

SERVINGS: 2

INGREDIENTS

- ½ cup avocado oil
- 1 small onion diced
- 1 tsp. garlic minced
- 1 cup pumpkin
- 1/4 cup fresh coriander washed.and chopped
- 1 cup crushed tomatoes

- 1 tbsp. tomato paste
- ½ tbsp. dried basil
- ½ tsp. salt and pepper

DIRECTIONS

1. Set the Instant Pot to Sauté. Add avocado oil and wait 1 minute to heat up.
2. Add the onion and garlic, sauté for 1 minute. Stir often.
3. Add the pumpkin, coriander, and sauté for 1 minute. Stir often.
4. Add the crushed tomatoes, tomato paste, dried basil, salt, and pepper. Stir well. Cover the Instant Pot and lock it in.
5. Set the Manual or Pressure Cook timer for 10 minutes. Make sure the timer is set to "Sealing".
6. Once the timer reaches zero, quickly release the pressure.
7. Enjoy!

NUTRITION

- Calories: 191
- Total Fat: 7. 6g
- Total Carbohydrate: 28. 9g

- Protein: 6g

EGGPLANT FETTUCCINE PASTA

PREPARATION TIME: **5 MIN**   COOKING TIME: **25 MIN**

SERVINGS: **2**

INGREDIENTS

- 1 tbsp. coconut oil
- 1 onion finely diced
- 1 medium zucchini chopped
- 2 cloves garlic minced
- 1 tbsp. tomato paste
- ½ cup vegetable broth
- 1 tsp. dried thyme
- 1 tsp. dried oregano

- 1 tsp. kosher salt
- ¼ tsp. pepper
- ½ cup diced tomatoes
- 1 cup eggplant, diced
- 1 tbsp. corn-starch
- 1 cup juice
- Shredded goat cheese for garnish

DIRECTIONS

1. Add coconut oil to the Instant Pot. Using the display panel select the Saute' function.
2. When oil gets hot, add onion to the Instant Pot and sauté for 3 minutes. Add zucchini and cook 3 minutes more. Add garlic and tomato paste and cook for 1-2 minutes more.
3. Add vegetable broth and seasonings to the Instant pot and deglaze by using a wooden spoon to scrape the brown bits from the bottom of the pot.
4. Add tomatoes to the Instant Pot and stir. Add eggplant to the Instant Pot, turning once to coat.
5. Turn the Instant pot off by selecting Cancel, then secure the lid, making sure the vent is closed.
6. Using the display panel select the Manual or Pressure Cook function. Use the +/- keys and program the Instant Pot for 20 minutes.
7. When the time is up, let the pressure naturally release for 15 minutes, then quickly release the remaining pressure.
8. In a small bowl, mix together 1/4 cup of Instant pot juices and corn-starch. Stir into the pot until thickened.
9. Serve hot topped with shredded cheese.

NUTRITION

- Calories: 405
- Total Fat: 14.2g
- Total Carbohydrate: 56.1g

- Dietary Fiber: 5.2g
- Protein: 16.1g

PASTA PUTTANESCA

PREPARATION TIME: 5 MIN   **COOKING TIME: 25 MIN**

SERVINGS: 2

INGREDIENTS

- 1 tsp. garlic powder
- ½ cup pasta sauce
- 2 cups water
- 2 cups dried rigatoni
- 1/4 cup crushed red pepper flakes
- ½ cup pitted Kalamata olives sliced
- ½ tsp. fine sea salt
- ¼ tsp. ground black pepper
- 1 tsp. grated lemon zest
- ½ cup broccoli

DIRECTIONS

1. Combine all of the ingredients in the inner cooking pot and stir to coat the pasta.
2. Lock the lid into place and turn the valve to "Sealing." Select Manual or Pressure Cook and adjust the pressure to High. Set the time for 5 minutes. When cooking ends, carefully turn the valve to "Venting" to quickly release the pressure. Unlock and remove the lid.
3. Serve hot.

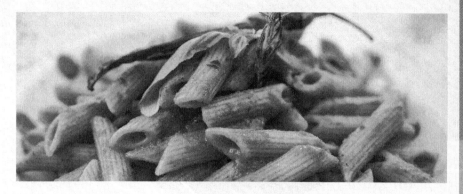

NUTRITION

- Calories: 383
- Total Fat: 4.2g
- Total Carbohydrate: 73.8g
- Dietary Fiber: 5g
- Protein: 12.4g

BASIL COCONUT PEAS AND BROCCOLI

PREPARATION TIME: **5 MIN**   COOKING TIME: **25 MIN**

SERVINGS: **2**

INGREDIENTS

- 1 cup coconut milk
- 1 cup basil
- 1 bell pepper seeded and cut into chunks
- 1 leek green part only, cut into chunks
- 1 tsp. garlic powder
- ¼ tsp. salt
- ½ cup water
- 1 cup noodles
- 1 cup green peas
- ½ cup broccoli florets

DIRECTIONS

1. In a blender add the coconut milk, basil, bell pepper, leek, garlic powder, and salt. Blend until smooth.
2. Pour the sauce into the inner pot and add the water. Select Sauté and adjust to High heat. Bring just to a simmer, then turn the Instant Pot off.
3. Break up the noodles into 3 or 4 pieces and place them in the pot in a single layer as much as possible. Layer the broccoli over the noodles.
4. Lock the lid into place. Select Pressure Cook or Manual, and adjust the pressure to Low and the time to 25 minutes. After cooking, quickly release the pressure.
5. Unlock the lid. Gently stir the mixture until the broccoli and peas are coated with sauce. Ladle into bowls and serve immediately.

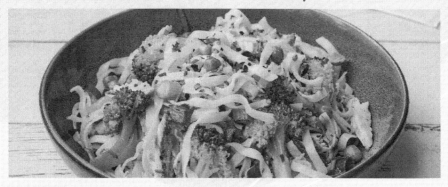

NUTRITION

- Calories: 499
- Total Fat: 31g
- Total Carbohydrate: 49.2g
- Dietary Fiber: 10g
- Protein: 12.8g

DINNER

BROWN RICE STIR FRY WITH VEGETABLES

PREPARATION TIME: 10 - 75 MIN   **COOKING TIME:** 25 MIN

SERVINGS: 4

INGREDIENTS

- 1 handful fresh parsley, chopped
- ½ zucchini, chopped
- 2 tbsp. olive oil
- 2 tbsp. soy sauce
- ½ bell pepper, chopped
- ½ cup brown rice, uncooked
- 4 garlic cloves, minced
- 1 cup red cabbage, chopped
- 1/8 tsp. cayenne powder
- ½ broccoli head, chopped
- Sesame seeds, for garnish

DIRECTIONS

1. Cook the brown rice as per the package instructions.
2. Bring water to a boil in a frying pan and then add veggies and make sure they are fully covered with water. Cook for 1-2 minutes on high heat, and then drain the water and set aside.
3. Add oil to the wok pan and heat over high heat and then add garlic along with parsley and cayenne powder. Cook for a minute stirring frequently and then add the drained veggies, tamari, and the cooked rice.
4. Cook for 1-2 minutes and then garnish with sesame seeds if desired. Serve and enjoy!

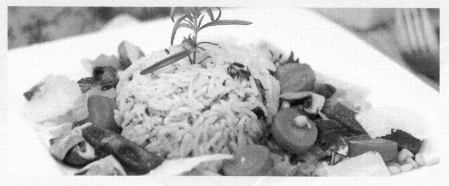

NUTRITION

- Calories: 140,
- Fat: 0.9g,
- Carbs: 27.1g,
- Protein: 6.3g,
- Fiber: 6.2g

GRILLED VEGGIE SKEWERS

PREPARATION TIME: 10 - 75 MIN   COOKING TIME: 15 MIN

SERVINGS: 4-6

INGREDIENTS

- 1 red onion, peeled, chopped
- 2 tbsp. avocado oil
- 2 portobello mushrooms, chopped
- 1 sweet potato, chopped
- 2 bell peppers, chopped
- 6 baby red potatoes, quartered
- Salt and black pepper, to taste
- 4 ears corn

DIRECTIONS

1. Preheat the oven to 375°F and add the sweet potato to a cooking pot along with the quartered potatoes and water. Bring to a boil and cook until lightly tender for about 10 minutes. When done, drain the water and let cool a bit.
2. Thread the vegetables onto skewers, and then brush them evenly with oil. When done, season the vegetables generously with salt and pepper on each side.
3. Cook the vegetables for about 10-15 minutes until tender and cooked through. Flip halfway. Place the corn directly on the vegetables to cook together.
4. When done, serve and enjoy with the desired sauce.

NUTRITION

- Calories: 680,
- Total Fat: 71.8g,
- Saturated Fat: 20.9g,
- Total Carbs: 10g,
- Dietary Fiber: 7g,
- Sugar: 2g,
- Protein: 3g,
- Sodium: 525mg

EGGPLANT TERIYAKI BOWLS

PREPARATION TIME: 10 - 75 MIN **COOKING TIME: 45 MIN**

SERVINGS: 4

INGREDIENTS

- 1 carrot, shredded
- 1 Chucky eggplant
- ¼ cup edamame beans, frozen
- 1 lime, ½ sliced, ½ juiced
- 2 spring onions, chopped
- 1½ tbsp. vegetable oil
- 1 handful radishes, sliced

- 1 tbsp. caster sugar
- 1 garlic clove, crushed
- ½ cup jasmine rice
- 2 tbsp. sesame seeds, toasted
- 1 small ginger, grated
- 2 tbsp. soy sauce

DIRECTIONS

1. Add 2 cups of water to a cooking pan, add rice and salt to taste. Bring to a boil, cook for a minute, and then close the lid. Reduce the heat to low and cook for 10 minutes until cooked through. Turn off the heat and steam for additional 10 minutes.
2. Add a tbsp. of oil to a bowl and toss the eggplant in it. Preheat the wok pan, add the eggplant, and cook for 5 minutes, stirring often, until lightly softened and charred. Add the carrots to the wok along with garlic, ginger, and spring onions, and then fry for 2-3 minutes.
3. In a small bowl, whisk the sugar along with soy sauce and a cup of water and then add into the wok. Simmer until the eggplant is very soft, for about 10-15 minutes.
4. Add water to the pan and bring to a boil and then add the frozen edamame beans, remove the beans, drain and rinse them well under running water. Add the radishes to a bowl, drain the beans again and then add them to the radishes. Squeeze lime juice on top and toss well until combined.
5. Serve the rice in the bowls and then scoop the eggplant and sauce on top along with the beans and radishes. Sprinkle with sesame seeds and garnish with lime slices. Enjoy

NUTRITION

- Calories: 140
- Fat: 0.9g
- Carbs: 27.1g

- Protein: 6.3g
- Fiber: 6.2g

QUINOA AND BLACK BEAN CHILI

PREPARATION TIME: 10 - 75 MIN   COOKING TIME: 45 MIN

SERVINGS: 8

INGREDIENTS

- 3 cups vegetable stock
- 1 onion, chopped
- 1 cup quinoa, rinsed, drained
- 1 red chili, chopped
- 2 tsp. ground cumin
- 1 lb. tomatoes, chopped
- olive oil spray

- 1 tsp. smoked paprika
- 1 small avocado, sliced
- ½ tsp. chili powder
- 2 garlic cloves, crushed
- 1 lb. black beans, rinsed, drained
- Coriander leaves, to serve

DIRECTIONS

1. Generously grease the cooking pan with oil and place over medium heat and then add the onion, red chili, and garlic. Fry the ingredients until soft, and then add spices and stir.
2. Add the vegetable stock into the pan along with quinoa, black beans, and tomatoes, and then adjust the seasonings if needed.
3. Close the lid and simmer until quinoa is tender, for about 30 minutes.
4. When done, garnish with coriander leaves and top with the avocado slices. Serve and enjoy!

NUTRITION

- Calories: 140,
- Fat: 0.9g,
- Carbs: 27.1g,

- Protein: 6.3g,
- Fiber: 6.2g

SNACK

ZUCCHINI HUMMUS

PREPARATION TIME: 5 MIN　　　　**COOKING TIME: 0 MIN**

SERVINGS: 8

INGREDIENTS

- 1 cup diced zucchini
- ½ tsp. sea salt
- 1 tsp. minced garlic
- 2 tsp. ground cumin
- 3 tbsp. lemon juice
- 1/3 cup tahini

DIRECTIONS

1. Place all the ingredients in a food processor and pulse for 2 minutes until smooth.
2. Tip the hummus in a bowl, drizzle with oil, and serve.

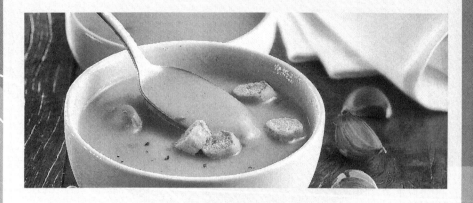

NUTRITION

- Calories: 65
- Fat: 5g
- Carbs: 3g
- Protein: 2g
- Fiber: 1g

CHIPOTLE AND LIME TORTILLA CHIPS

PREPARATION TIME: **10 MIN**   COOKING TIME: **15 MIN**

SERVINGS: **4**

INGREDIENTS

- 12 oz. whole-wheat tortillas
- 4 tbsp. chipotle seasoning 1 tbsp. olive oil
- 4 limes, juiced

DIRECTIONS

1. Whisk together oil and lime juice, brush it well on tortillas, then sprinkle with chipotle seasoning and bake for 15 minutes at 350° F until crispy, turning halfway.
2. When done, let the tortilla cool for 10 minutes, then break it into chips and serve.

NUTRITION

- Calories: 150
- Fat: 7g
- Carbs: 18g

- Protein: 2g
- Fiber: 2g

CARROT AND SWEET POTATO FRITTERS

PREPARATION TIME: **10 MIN**   COOKING TIME: **8 MIN**

SERVINGS: **10**

INGREDIENTS

- 1/3 cup quinoa flour
- 1½ cups shredded sweet potato
- 1 cup grated carrot
- 1/3 tsp. ground black pepper
- 2/3 tsp. salt
- 2 tsp. curry powder
- 2 flax eggs

- 2 tbsp. coconut oil

DIRECTIONS

1. Place all the ingredients in a bowl, except for oil, stir well until combined, and then shape the mixture into ten small patties
2. Take a large pan, place it over medium-high heat, add oil and when it melts, add patties in it and cook for 3 minutes per side until browned.
3. Serve straight away

NUTRITION

- Calories: 70
- Fat: 3g
- Carbs: 8g

- Protein: 1g
- Fiber: 1g

CHAPTER 8
VEGAN RECIPES - BREAKFAST

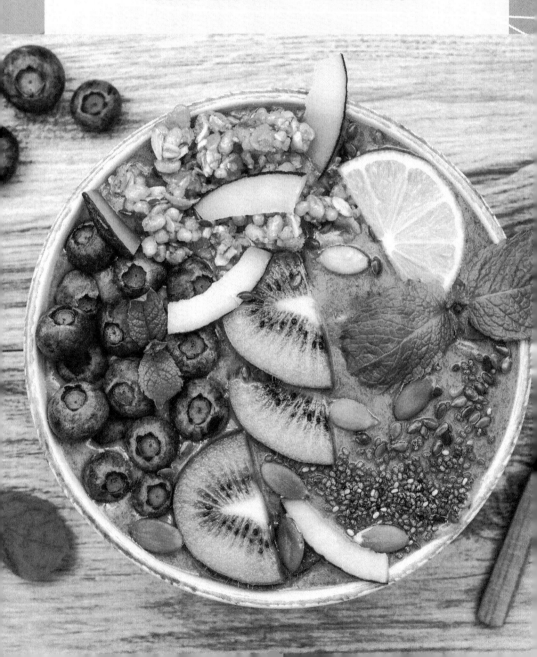

VEGAN BREAKFAST HASH

PREPARATION TIME: **15-30 MIN**   COOKING TIME: **25 MIN**

SERVINGS: **4**

INGREDIENTS

- 1 Bell Pepper
- ½ tsp. Smoked Paprika
- 3 medium potatoes
- 8 oz. Mushrooms
- 1 Yellow Onion
- 1 Zucchini
- ½ tsp. Cumin Powder
- ½ tsp. Garlic Powder
- Salt and Pepper
- 2 tbsp. Cooking oil (optional

DIRECTIONS

1. Heat a large pan on medium fflame, add oil, and put the sliced potatoes
2. Cook the potatoes till they change color
3. Cut the rest of the vegetables and add all the spices
4. Cooked till veggies are soften

NUTRITION

- Carbs: 29. 7g
- Protein: 5. 5g
- Fat: 10g
- Calories: 217

VEGAN MUFFINS BREAKFAST SANDWICH

PREPARATION TIME: 15-30 MIN   **COOKING TIME: 20 MIN**

SERVINGS: 2

INGREDIENTS

- 3-4 tbsp. Romesco Sauce
- ½ cup Fresh baby spinach
- 2 Tofu Scramble
- 2 Vegan English muffins
- ½ peeled and sliced Avocado
- 1 Sliced fresh tomato

DIRECTIONS

1. In the oven, toast English muffin
2. Half the muffin and spread romesco sauce
3. Paste spinach to 1 side, tailed by avocado slices
4. Have warm tofu followed by a tomato slice
5. Place the other muffin half onto the preceding one

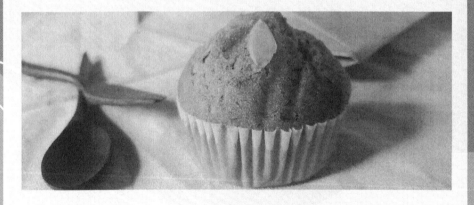

NUTRITION

- Carbs: 18g
- Protein: 12g
- Fat: 14g

- Calories: 276

ALMOND WAFFLES WITH CRANBERRIES

PREPARATION TIME: 15-30 MIN   **COOKING TIME: 20 MIN**

SERVINGS: 4

INGREDIENTS

- 2 tbsp. flax seed powder + 6 tbsp. water
- 2/3 cup almond flour
- 2½ tsp. baking powder
- A pinch of salt
- 1½ cups almond milk
- 2 tbsp. plant butter
- 1 cup fresh almond butter
- 2 tbsp. pure maple syrup
- 1 tsp. fresh lemon juice

DIRECTIONS

1. In a medium bowl, mix the flax seed powder with water and allow soaking for 5 minutes.
2. Add the almond flour, baking powder, salt, and almond milk. Mix until well combined.
3. Preheat a waffle iron and brush with some plant butter. Pouruntil the waffles are golden and crisp, 2 to 3 minutes.
4. Transfer the waffles to a plate and make more waffles using the same process and ingredient proportions.
5. Meanwhile, in a medium bowl, mix the almond butter with maple syrup mixture, and serve.

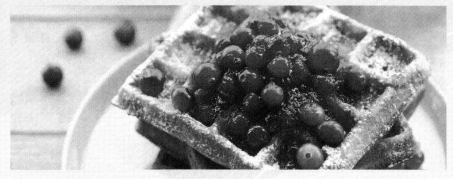

NUTRITION

- Calories: 533
- Fat: 53g
- Carbs: 16.7g
- Protein: 1.2g

CHICKPEA OMELET WITH SPINACH AND MUSHROOMS

PREPARATION TIME: 5-15 MIN   **COOKING TIME: 25 MIN**

SERVINGS: 4

INGREDIENTS

- 1 cup chickpea flour
- ½ tsp. onion powder
- ½ tsp. garlic powder
- ¼ tsp. white pepper
- ¼ tsp. black pepper
- 1/3 cup nutritional yeast
- ½ tsp. baking soda
- 1 small green bell pepper, deseeded and chopped
- 3 scallions, chopped
- 1 cup sautéed sliced white button mushrooms
- ½ cup chopped fresh spinach
- 1 cup halved cherry tomatoes for serving
- 1 tbsp. fresh parsley leaves

DIRECTIONS

1. In a medium bowl, mix the chickpea flour, onion powder, garlic powder, white pepper, black pepper, nutritional yeast, and baking soda until well combined.
2. Heat a medium skillet over medium heat and add a quarter of the batter. Swirl the pan to spread the batter across the pan. Scatter a quarter each of the bell pepper, scallions, mushrooms, and spinach on top, and cook until the bottom part of the omelet sets and is golden brown, 1 to 2 minutes. Carefully, flip the omelet and cook the other side until set and golden brown.
3. Transfer the omelet to a plate and make the remaining omelets using the remaining batter in the same proportions.
4. Serve the omelet with the tomatoes and garnish with the parsley leaves.

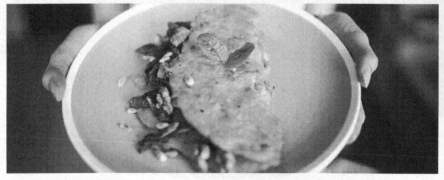

NUTRITION

- Calories: 147,
- Fat: 1.8g,
- Carbs: 21.3g,
- Protein: 11.6g

LUNCH

ROASTED VEGETABLES

PREPARATION TIME: 15 MIN   **COOKING TIME: 40 MIN**

SERVINGS: 4

INGREDIENTS

- ¼ summer squash, cubed
- 1 red bell peppers, seeded and diced
- 1 red onion, quartered
- ¼ cup green beans
- 1 tbsp. chopped fresh thyme
- 2 tbsp. chopped fresh rosemary
- ¼ cup olive oil
- ½ tbsp. lemon juice
- Salt and freshly ground black pepper

DIRECTIONS

1. Preheat oven to 475° F.
2. In a large bowl, combine the squash, red bell peppers, and green beans. Separate the red onion quarters into pieces, and add them to the mixture.
3. In a small bowl, stir together thyme, rosemary, olive oil, lemon juice, salt, and pepper. Toss with vegetables until they are coated. Spread evenly on a large roasting pan.
4. Roast for 35 to 40 minutes in the preheated oven, stirring every 10 minutes, or until vegetables are cooked through and browned.

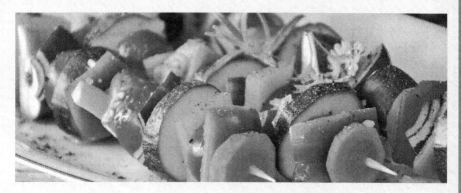

NUTRITION

- Calories: 145,
- Total Fat: 13.1g,
- Saturated Fat: 2g,
- Cholesterol: 0mg,
- Sodium: 4mg,
- Total Carbohydrate: 8g,
- Dietary Fiber: 2.5g,
- Total Sugars: 3.5g,
- Protein: 1.3g,
- Calcium: 47mg,
- Iron: 2mg,
- Potassium: 160mg,
- Phosphorus: 110mg

HONEY ROASTED CAULIFLOWER

PREPARATION TIME: 10 MIN   **COOKING TIME: 35 MIN**

SERVINGS: 4

INGREDIENTS

- 2 cups cauliflower
- 2 tbsp. diced onion
- 2 tbsp. olive oil
- 1 tbsp. honey
- 1 tsp. dry mustard
- 1 pinch of salt
- 1 pinch ground black pepper

DIRECTIONS

1. Preheat oven to 375° F. Lightly coat an 11x7 inch baking dish with non-stick cooking spray.
2. Place cauliflower in a single layer in the prepared dish, and top with onion. In a small bowl, combine olive oil, honey, mustard, salt, and pepper; drizzle over cauliflower and onion.
3. Bake in the preheated 375° F oven for 35 minutes or until tender, stirring halfway through the cooking time.

NUTRITION

- Calories: 88
- Total Fat: 7.3g
- Total Carbohydrate: 6.4g
- Dietary Fiber: 0.9g
- Protein: 0.8g

BROCCOLI STEAKS

PREPARATION TIME: **10 MIN**   COOKING TIME: **25 MIN**

SERVINGS: **4**

INGREDIENTS

- 1 medium head broccoli
- 3 tbsp. unsalted butter
- ¼ tsp. garlic powder
- ¼ tsp. onion powder
- 1/8 tsp. salt
- ¼ tsp. pepper

DIRECTIONS

1. Preheat the oven to 400° F. Please parchment paper on a roasting pan.
2. Trim the leaves off the broccoli and cut off the bottom of the stem. Cut the broccoli head in half. Cut each half into 1 to 3/4-inch slices, leaving the core in place. Cut off the smaller ends of the broccoli and save for another recipe. There should be 4 broccoli steaks.
3. Mix butter, garlic powder, onion powder, salt, and pepper.
4. Lay the broccoli on the parchment-lined baking sheet. Using half of the butter mixture, brush onto the steaks. Place in the preheated oven for 20 remaining butter and roast for about 20 more minutes, until they are golden brown on the edges.

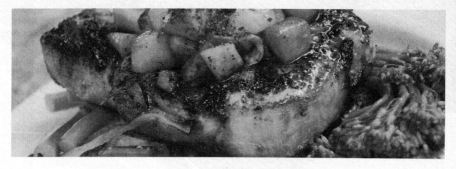

NUTRITION

- Calories: 86
- Total Fat: 8.7g
- Total Carbohydrate: 1.9g
- Dietary Fiber: 0.7g
- Protein: 0.8g

DINNER

BUTTERNUT SQUASH RISOTTO

PREPARATION TIME: **20 MIN**   COOKING TIME: **15-120 MIN**

SERVINGS: **8**

INGREDIENTS

- 3 tbsp. extra virgin olive oil
- 1½ oz. butternut squash, peeled, halved, seeds removed and cubed
- 2 tsp. ground sage
- Sea salt and black pepper
- 1 onion, diced
- 5½ cups vegetable broth

- 4 tbsp. vegan butter
- 2½ cups arborio rice
- 1 cup dry white wine (optional)
- 1 tbsp. nutritional yeast (optional)

DIRECTIONS

1. On saute feature, heat olive oil and add squash, sage, salt, and pepper.
2. Cook for 9 minutes.
3. Add onion and cook for 1 minute. Add vegan butter, wine (optional), and broth. Stir to combine. Add rice and stir.
4. Close the lid and seal. On manual mode, set time to 5 minutes.
5. When done, quick release. Stir in the nutritional yeast and allow to sit for 5 minutes to thicken.
6. Serve warm. Enjoy!

NUTRITION

- Calories: 140,
- Fat: 0.9g,
- Carbs: 27.1g,

- Protein: 6.3g,
- Fiber: 6.2g

SWEET POTATOES

PREPARATION TIME: **29 MIN**   COOKING TIME: **15-120 MIN**

SERVINGS: **4**

INGREDIENTS

- 4 Sweet Potatoes, scrubbed and rinsed
- 1½ Cups Water

OPTIONAL TOPPINGS:
- Scrambled Tofu, Avocado, Tomatoes
- Vegan Butter, Coconut Sugar, Cinnamon
- Arugula, Olive Oil, Lemon, Sea Salt

DIRECTIONS

1. Add water to the instant pot.
2. Place the steaming tray inside and put potatoes on top.
3. Cover with lid and seal.
4. Pressure cook for 18 minutes on manual mode.
5. When done cooking, allow pressure to release on its own (about 15 minutes).
6. Remove lid.
7. Serve immediately with desired toppings. Enjoy!

NUTRITION

- Calories: 140
- Fat: 0.9g
- Carbs: 27.1g
- Protein: 6.3g
- Fiber: 6.2g

THAI GREEN CURRY WITH SPRING VEGETABLES

PREPARATION TIME: 10-75 MIN   **COOKING TIME:** 45 MIN

SERVINGS: 4

INGREDIENTS

- 1 cup brown basmati rice or rice noodles, rinsed
- 2 tsp. coconut oil
- 1 onion, diced
- 1 tbsp. fresh ginger, chopped
- 2 cloves garlic, chopped
- 2 cups asparagus, sliced
- 1 cup carrots, peeled and sliced
- 2 tbsp. Thai green curry paste
- 14 oz. full-fat coconut milk (I used full-fat coconut milk for a more decadent curry)
- ½ cup water
- 1½ tsp. coconut sugar
- 2 cups packed baby spinach, chopped
- 1½ tsp. fresh lime juice
- 1½ tsp. tamari
- salt

DIRECTIONS

1. Place a pot over medium heat. Add water and bring it to a boil.
2. Add rice, salt to taste and cook for 30 minutes. When done, cover the rice and set aside for more than 10 minutes.
3. Place a large skillet over medium heat. Add oil.
4. Cook onion, garlic, ginger, and a pinch of salt. Add asparagus, carrots and cook for 3 minutes. Add curry paste and cook for additional 2 minutes.
5. Add coconut milk, ½ cup water, sugar and bring this mixture to a simmer. Reduce the heat and let it cook for 10 minutes until vegetables are tender.
6. Add spinach and let it cook for ½ a minute. Remove from the heat and season with rice vinegar and tamari.

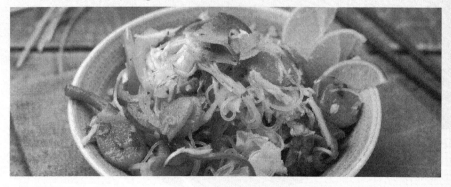

NUTRITION

- Calories: 140,
- Fat: 0.9g,
- Carbs: 27.1g,
- Protein: 6.3g,
- Fiber: 6.2g

SNACK

POLENTA SKEWERS

PREPARATION TIME: 35 MIN   **COOKING TIME: 0 MIN**

SERVINGS: 4

INGREDIENTS

- ½ avocado
- 10 cherry tomatoes
- 1 mini zucchini
- 150g. corn grits
- 2 tbsp. olive oil
- 1 tsp. sesame seeds, black
- 10 basil leaves
- 10 toothpicks
- 450 ml vegetable stock
- Salt and pepper

DIRECTIONS

1. The day before, bring the corn grits to the boil in the broth and cook for a few minutes, stirring constantly. Pour into a square form and chill until the next day.
2. Cut the polenta into small cubes and fry in a pan in a little olive oil.
3. Wash the zucchini, cut into thin slices, and fry in the pan once the polenta is ready. Wash the tomatoes and cut them in half, pluck the basil leaves from the branches.
4. Stone the avocado and cut into thin slices.
5. Skewer a polenta cube, a zucchini, a tomato, a slice of avocado, and a basil leaf onto a toothpick. Serve with sesame seeds.

NUTRITION

- Calories: 259
- Fat: 15.4g
- Carbs: 20.5g
- Protein: 12.1g
- Fiber: 3.2g

BOREK WITH SPINACH FILLING

PREPARATION TIME: 25 MIN   **COOKING TIME: 20 MIN**

SERVINGS: 10

INGREDIENTS

- 10 yufka sheets
- 2 cloves of garlic
- 1 small onion
- 3 tbsp. soy yogurt
- 4 tbsp. soy milk
- 400g. spin nat
- 3 tbsp. of oil
- 1 pinch of nutmeg
- Salt and pepper

DIRECTIONS

1. Wash the spinach, peel the garlic and onion and cut into small cubes.
2. Steam the spinach, onion, and garlic in oil in a deep pan.
3. After a few minutes, season with nutmeg, salt, and pepper and stir in the yogurt.
4. Layout the Yufka leaves and brush with the spinach filling.
5. Roll up and brush with a bit of milk.
6. Then place on a baking sheet and bake in the oven at 180° C for about 15 minutes.

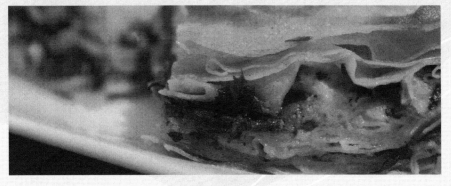

NUTRITION

- Calories: 219
- Fat: 9.4g
- Carbs: 10.5g
- Protein: 11.1g
- Fiber: 3.2g

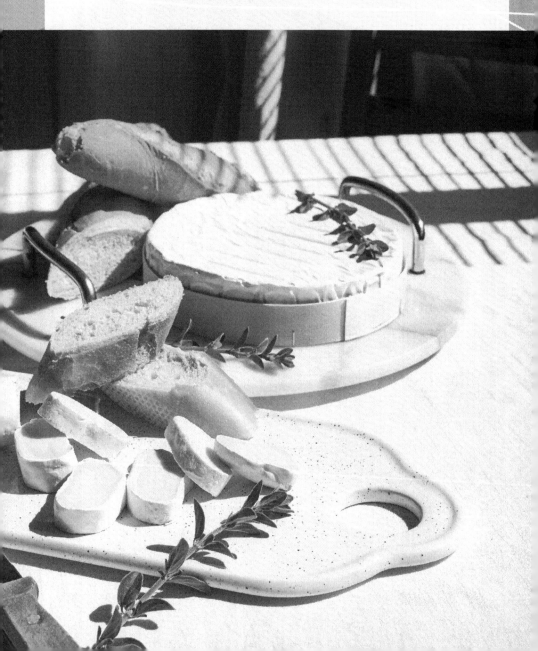

CHAPTER 9
MEDITERRANEAN RECIPES - BREAKFAST

QUINOA FRUIT SALAD

PREPARATION TIME: 25 MIN   **COOKING TIME: 0 MIN**

SERVINGS: 4

INGREDIENTS

- 2 tablespoons honey, raw
- 1 cup strawberries, fresh & sliced
- 2 tablespoons lime juice, fresh
- 1 teaspoon basil, fresh & chopped
- 1 cup quinoa, cooked
- 1 mango, peeled, pitted & diced
- 1 cup blackberries, fresh
- 1 peach, pitted & diced
- 2 kiwis, peeled & quartered

DIRECTIONS

1. Start by mixing your lime juice, basil and honey together in a small bowl. In a different bowl mix your strawberries, quinoa, blackberries, peach, kiwis and mango. Add in your honey mixture, and toss to coat before serving.

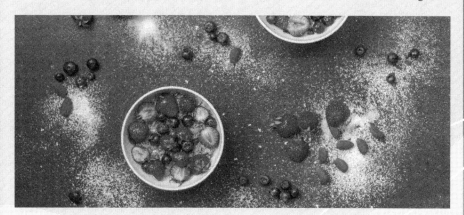

NUTRITION

- 159 calories
- 12g fats
- 29g protein

STRAWBERRY RHUBARB SMOOTHIE

PREPARATION TIME: **8 MIN**   COOKING TIME: **0 MIN**

SERVINGS: **1**

INGREDIENTS

- 1 cup strawberries, fresh & sliced
- 1 rhubarb stalk, chopped
- 2 tablespoons honey, raw
- 3 ice cubes
- 1/8 teaspoon ground cinnamon
- ½ cup Greek yogurt, plain

DIRECTIONS

1. Start by getting out a small saucepan and fill it with water. Place it over high heat to bring it to a boil, and then add in your rhubarb. Boil for three minutes before draining and transferring it to a blender.
2. In your blender add in your yogurt, honey, cinnamon and strawberries. Blend until smooth, and then add in your ice. Blend until there are no lumps and it's thick. Enjoy cold.

NUTRITION

- 201 calories
- 11g fats
- 39g protein

BUCKWHEAT BUTTERMILK PANCAKES

PREPARATION TIME: **2 MIN**   COOKING TIME: **18 MIN**

SERVINGS: **9**

INGREDIENTS

- ½ cup of buckwheat flour
- ½ cup of all-purpose flour
- 2 teaspoons of baking powder
- 1 teaspoon of brown sugar
- 2 tablespoons of olive oil
- 2 large eggs
- 1 cup of reduced-fat buttermilk

DIRECTIONS

1.   Combine the first four ingredients in a bowl. Add the oil, buttermilk, and eggs and mix until thoroughly blended.
2.   Place a skillet or griddle over medium heat and spray with non-stick cooking spray.
3.   Pour ¼ cup of the batter over the skillet and cook for 1-2 minutes each side or until they turn golden brown. Serve immediately.

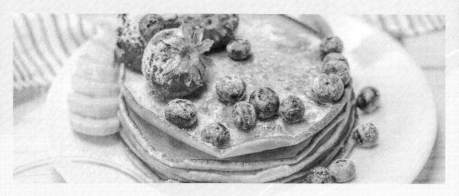

NUTRITION

- 108 Calories
- 12g Carbohydrates
- 1g Fiber

- 4g Protein

FRENCH TOAST WITH ALMONDS AND PEACH COMPOTE

PREPARATION TIME: **10 MIN**   COOKING TIME: **15 MIN**

SERVINGS: **4**

INGREDIENTS

- 3 tablespoons of sugar substitute, sucralose-based
- 1/3 cup + 2 tablespoons of water, divided
- 1 and 1/2 cups of fresh peeled or frozen, thawed and drained sliced peaches
- 2 tablespoons peach fruit spread, no-sugar-added
- 1/4 teaspoon of ground cinnamon
- Almond French toast

- 1/4 cup of (skim) fat-free milk
- 3 tablespoons of sugar substitute, sucralose-based
- 2 whole eggs
- 2 egg whites
- 1/2 teaspoon of almond extract
- 1/8 teaspoon salt
- 4 slices of multigrain bread
- 1/3 cup of sliced almonds

DIRECTIONS

1. To make the compote, dissolve 3 tablespoons sucralose in 1/3 cup of water in a medium saucepan over high-medium heat. Stir in the peaches and bring to a boil. Reduce the heat to medium and continue to cook uncovered for another 5 minutes or until the peaches softened.
2. Combine remaining water and fruit spread then stir into the peaches in the saucepan. Cook for another minute or until syrup thickens. Remove from heat and stir in the cinnamon. Cover to keep warm.
3. To make the French toast. Combine the milk and sucralose in a large size shallow dish and whisk until it completely dissolves. Whisk in the egg whites, eggs, almond extract and salt. Dip both sides of the bread slices for 3 minutes in the egg mixture or until completely soaked. Sprinkle both sides with sliced almonds and press firmly to adhere.
4. Spray a non-stick skillet or griddle with cooking spray and place over medium-high heat. Cook bread slices on griddle for 2 to 3 minutes both sides or until it turns light brown. Serve topped with the peach compote.

NUTRITION

- 277 Calories
- 31g Carbohydrates
- 7g Fiber

- 12g Protein

MIXED BERRIES OATMEAL WITH SWEET VANILLA CREAM

PREPARATION TIME: **5 MIN**   COOKING TIME: **5 MIN**

SERVINGS: **4**

INGREDIENTS

- 2 cups water
- 1 cup of quick-cooking oats
- 1 tablespoon of sucralose-based sugar substitute
- 1/2 teaspoon of ground cinnamon
- 1/8 teaspoon salt

CREAM
- 3/4 cup of fat-free half-and-half
- 3 tablespoons of sucralose-based sugar substitute

- 1/2 teaspoon of vanilla extract
- 1/2 teaspoon of almond extract

TOPPINGS
- 1- 1/2 cups of fresh or frozen and thawed blueberries
- 1/2 cup of fresh or frozen and thawed raspberries

DIRECTIONS

1. Boil water in high-heat and stir in the oats. Reduce heat to medium while cooking oats, uncovered for 2 minutes or until thick.
2. Remove from heat and stir in sugar substitute, salt and cinnamon. In a medium size bowl, combine all the cream ingredients until well blended. Scoop cooked oatmeal into 4 equal portions and pour the sweet cream over. Top with the berries and serve.

NUTRITION

- 150 Calories
- 30g Carbohydrates
- 5g Fiber

- 5g Protein

MEDITERRANEAN PITA BREAKFAST

PREPARATION TIME: **22 MIN**   COOKING TIME: **3 MIN**

SERVINGS: **2**

INGREDIENTS

- 1/4 cup of sweet red pepper, chopped
- 1/4 cup of chopped onion
- 1 cup of egg substitute
- 1/8 teaspoon of salt
- 1/8 teaspoon of pepper
- 1 small chopped tomato
- 1/2 cup of fresh torn baby spinach
- 1-1/2 teaspoons of minced fresh basil
- 2 whole size pita breads
- 2 tablespoons of crumbled feta cheese

DIRECTIONS

1. Coat with a cooking spray a small size non-stick skillet. Stir in the onion and red pepper for 3 minutes over medium heat.
2. Add your egg substitute and season with salt and pepper. Stir cook until it sets. Mix the torn spinach, chopped tomatoes, and mince basil. Scoop onto the pitas.
3. Top vegetable mixture with your egg mixture. Sprinkle with crumbled feta cheese and serve immediately.

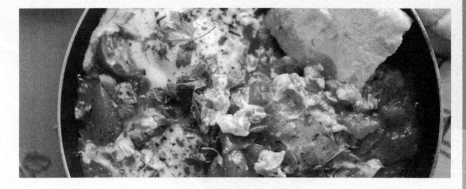

NUTRITION

- 267 Calories
- 41g Carbohydrates
- 3g Fiber
- 20g Protein

LUNCH

PASTA WITH PESTO

PREPARATION TIME: **10 MIN**   COOKING TIME: **0 MIN**

SERVINGS: **4**

INGREDIENTS

- 3 tablespoons extra-virgin olive oil
- 3 garlic cloves, finely minced
- ½ cup fresh basil leaves
- ¼ cup (about 2 ounces) grated Parmesan or Pecorino cheese
- ¼ cup pine nuts

- 8 ounces whole-wheat pasta, cooked according to package instructions and drained

DIRECTIONS

1. In a blender or food processor, combine the olive oil, garlic, basil, cheese, and pine nuts. Pulse for 10 to 20 (1-second) pulses until everything is chopped and blended.
2. Toss with the hot pasta and serve.

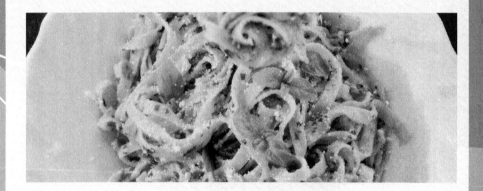

NUTRITION

- Calories: 405;
- Protein: 13g;
- Total Carbohydrates: 44g;

- Sugars: 2g;
- Fiber: 5g;
- Total Fat: 21g;

CHEESY CAPRESE SALAD SKEWERS

PREPARATION TIME: 15 MIN   **COOKING TIME: 0 MIN**

SERVINGS: 10

INGREDIENTS

- 8-oz cherry tomatoes, sliced in half
- A handful of fresh basil leaves, rinsed and drained
- 1-lb fresh mozzarella, cut into bite-sized slices
- Balsamic vinegar
- Extra virgin olive oil
- Freshly ground black pepper
- Toothpicks

DIRECTIONS

1. Sandwich a folded basil leaf and mozzarella cheese between the halves of tomato onto a toothpick.
2. Drizzle with olive oil and balsamic vinegar each skewer. To serve, sprinkle with freshly ground black pepper.

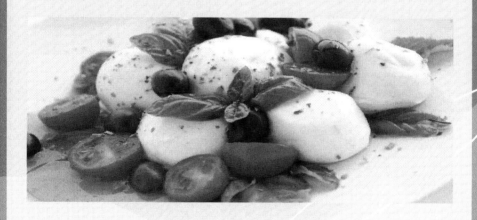

NUTRITION

- Calories: 94
- Total Fats: 3.7g
- Fiber: 2g
- Carbohydrates: 15.4g
- Protein: 2.1g

MEDITERRANEAN INSTANT POT SHREDDED BEEF

PREPARATION TIME: **5 MIN**   COOKING TIME: **25 MIN**

SERVINGS: **8**

INGREDIENTS

- 2 pounds Chuck beef roast
- 1 teaspoon salt
- 1 cup white onion, chopped
- ¾ cup carrots, chopped
- ¾ cup yellow bell pepper, chopped
- 14.5 ounce can of fire-roasted tomatoes
- 2 tablespoons red wine vinegar
- 1 tablespoon garlic, minced
- 1 tablespoon Italian seasoning blend
- 1/2 tablespoon dried red pepper flakes

DIRECTIONS

1. Cut the beef roast into small chunks, and trim away any excess fat. Season with salt.
2. Place the small beef cubes into the instant pot and then top with onions, carrots, and yellow bell peppers.
3. Open the can of fire-roasted tomatoes and stir in the vinegar, garlic, Italian dressing, and red pepper flakes. Pour mixture over the beef in the instant pot.
4. Secure the lid and set the vent to sealed. Set for 20 minutes on the high-pressure setting.
5. When the timer goes off, quick release to remove pressure, remove lid carefully, and let stand for 5-10 minutes. Use a large fork to shred beef into bite-sized pieces and then serve.

NUTRITION

- Calories: 190.2
- Protein: 23.5 g
- Total Fat: 6.3 g
- Carbohydrates: 8.9 g

PASTA WITH CREAMY TOMATO SAUCE

PREPARATION TIME: 10 MIN   **COOKING TIME: 10 MIN**

SERVINGS: 4

INGREDIENTS

- 16 ounces linguine
- 2 cups chopped onion
- 1 cup chopped carrot
- ½ cup dry white wine
- ½ cup raw unsalted cashew pieces
- ¼ to ½ cup of water
- 2 (14.5-ounce) cans diced tomatoes
- 4 garlic cloves, peeled
- 24 large basil leaves, 12 left whole and 12 cut into thin ribbons
- 1 teaspoon of sea salt
- ¼ teaspoon freshly ground black pepper

DIRECTIONS

1. Bring a large pot of water to a boil over high heat and cook the pasta until al dente according to the directions on the package. Drain.
2. Meanwhile, in a large skillet, combine the onion, carrot, and wine. (If you're not using a high-speed blender, add the cashews now as well.) Sauté the vegetables over medium heat for 5 minutes, stirring often. As you go, add the water, as needed, to prevent sticking.
3. Add the tomatoes and their juices. Cook, often stirring, for another 5 minutes.
4. Transfer the mixture to a high-speed blender. Add the garlic, whole basil leaves, cashews, salt, and pepper. Blend until very smooth.
5. Serve generous portions of the sauce over the pasta and top with the fresh basil ribbons.

NUTRITION

- Calories: 532;
- Total Fat: 11g;
- Saturated Fat: 2g;
- Protein: 17g;
- Carbohydrates: 85g;
- Fiber: 8g;

SHRIMPS WITH LEMON AND PEPPER

PREPARATION TIME: 10 MIN   **COOKING TIME: 3 MIN**

SERVINGS: 4

INGREDIENTS

- 40 big shrimp, peeled and deveined
- 6 garlic cloves, minced
- Salt and black pepper to taste
- 3 tablespoons olive oil
- ¼ teaspoon sweet paprika
- A pinch of red pepper flakes, crushed
- ¼ teaspoon lemon zest, grated
- 3 tablespoons sherry
- 1 and ½ tablespoons chives, sliced
- Juice of 1 lemon

DIRECTIONS

1. Heat a pan with the oil over medium high heat, add shrimp, season with salt and pepper and cook for 1 minute.
2. Add paprika, garlic and pepper flakes, stir and cook for 1 minute.
3. Add sherry, stir and cook for 1 minute more.
4. Take shrimp off heat, add chives and lemon zest, stir and transfer shrimp to plates. Add lemon juice all over and serve.

NUTRITION

- Calories 140
- Fat 1g
- Fiber 0g
- Carbs 1g
- Protein 18g

DINNER

TUNA AND POTATO SALAD

PREPARATION TIME: 10 MIN　　　**COOKING TIME: NIL**

SERVINGS: 4

INGREDIENTS

- 1 pound baby potatoes, scrubbed, boiled
- 1 cup tuna chunks, drained
- 1 cup cherry tomatoes, halved
- 1 cup medium onion, thinly sliced
- 8 pitted black olives
- 2 medium hard-boiled eggs, sliced
- 1 head Romaine lettuce
- Honey lemon mustard dressing
- ¼ cup olive oil
- 2 tablespoons lemon juice
- 1 tablespoon Dijon mustard
- 1 teaspoon dill weed, chopped
- Salt as needed
- Pepper as needed

DIRECTIONS

1. Take a small glass bowl and mix in your olive oil, honey, lemon juice, Dijon mustard and dill.
2. Season the mix with pepper and salt.
3. Add in the tuna, baby potatoes, cherry tomatoes, red onion, green beans, black olives and toss. everything nicely.
4. Arrange your lettuce leaves on a beautiful serving dish to make the base of your salad.
5. Top them with your salad mixture and place the egg slices.
6. Drizzle it with the previously prepared Salad Dressing. Serve hot.

NUTRITION

- Calories: 406
- Fat: 22g
- Carbohydrates: 28g
- Protein: 26g

BAKED ORZO WITH EGGPLANT, SWISS CHARD, AND MOZZARELLA

PREPARATION TIME: 20 MIN   **COOKING TIME: 1 HOUR**

SERVINGS: 4

INGREDIENTS

- 2 tablespoons extra-virgin olive oil
- 1 large (1-pound) eggplant, diced small
- 2 carrots, peeled and diced small
- 2 celery stalks, diced small
- 1 onion, diced small
- ½ teaspoon kosher salt
- 3 garlic cloves, minced
- ¼ teaspoon freshly ground black pepper
- 1 cup whole-wheat orzo
- 1 teaspoon no-salt-added tomato paste
- 1½ cups no-salt-added vegetable stock
- 1 cup Swiss chard, stemmed and chopped small
- 2 tablespoons fresh oregano, chopped
- Zest of 1 lemon
- 4 ounces mozzarella cheese, diced small
- ¼ cup grated Parmesan cheese
- 2 tomatoes, sliced ½-inch-thick

DIRECTIONS

1. Preheat the oven to 400°F. Heat the olive oil in a large oven-safe sauté pan over medium heat.
2. Add the eggplant, carrots, celery, onion, and salt and sauté about 10 minutes. Add the garlic and black pepper and sauté about 30 seconds. Add the orzo and tomato paste and sauté 1 minute. Add the vegetable stock and deglaze the pan, scraping up the brown bits. Add the Swiss chard, oregano, and lemon zest and stir until the chard wilts.
3. Remove from the heat and mix in the mozzarella cheese. Smooth the top of the orzo mixture flat. Sprinkle the Parmesan cheese over the top
4. .Arrange the tomatoes in a single layer on top of the Parmesan cheese. Bake for 45 minutes.

NUTRITION

- 470 Calories
- 17g Total fat
- 7g Fiber
- 18g Protein

BARLEY RISOTTO WITH TOMATOES

PREPARATION TIME: 20 MIN   **COOKING TIME: 45 MIN**

SERVINGS: 4

INGREDIENTS

- 2 tablespoons extra-virgin olive oil
- 2 celery stalks, diced
- ½ cup shallots, diced
- 4 garlic cloves, minced
- 3 cups no-salt-added vegetable stock
- 1 (14.5-ounce) can no-salt-added diced tomatoes
- 1 (14.5-ounce) can no-salt-added crushed tomatoes
- 1 cup pearl barley
- Zest of 1 lemon

- 1 teaspoon kosher salt
- ½ teaspoon smoked paprika
- ¼ teaspoon red pepper flakes
- ¼ teaspoon freshly ground black pepper
- 4 thyme sprigs
- 1 dried bay leaf
- 2 cups baby spinach
- ½ cup crumbled feta cheese
- 1 tablespoon fresh oregano, chopped
- 1 tablespoon fennel seeds, toasted (optional)

DIRECTIONS

1. Heat the olive oil in a large saucepan over medium heat. Add the celery and shallots and sauté, about 4 to 5 minutes. Add the garlic and sauté 30 seconds.
2. Add the vegetable stock, diced tomatoes, crushed tomatoes, barley, lemon zest, salt, paprika, red pepper flakes, black pepper, thyme, and the bay leaf, and mix well. Bring to a boil, then lower to low, and simmer. Cook, stirring occasionally, for 40 minutes.
3. Remove the bay leaf and thyme sprigs. Stir in the spinach. In a small bowl, combine the feta, oregano, and fennel seeds. Serve the barley risotto in bowls topped with the feta mixture.

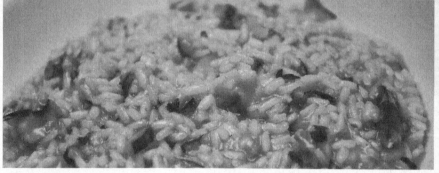

NUTRITION

- 375 Calories
- 12g Total fat

- 13g Fiber
- 11g Protein

CHICKPEAS AND KALE WITH SPICY POMODORO SAUCE

PREPARATION TIME: 10 MIN   **COOKING TIME: 35 MIN**

SERVINGS: 4

INGREDIENTS

- 2 tablespoons extra-virgin olive oil
- 4 garlic cloves, sliced
- 1 teaspoon red pepper flakes
- 1 (28-ounce) can no-salt-added crushed tomatoes
- 1 teaspoon kosher salt
- ½ teaspoon honey
- 1 bunch kale, stemmed and chopped
- 2 (15-ounce) cans low-sodium chickpeas, drained and rinsed
- ¼ cup fresh basil, chopped
- ¼ cup grated pecorino Romano cheese

DIRECTIONS

1. Heat the olive oil in a large skillet or sauté pan over medium heat. Add the garlic and red pepper flakes and sauté until the garlic is a light golden brown, about 2 minutes. Add the tomatoes, salt, and honey and mix well. Reduce the heat to low and simmer for 20 minutes.
2. Add the kale and mix in well. Cook about 5 minutes. Add the chickpeas and simmer about 5 minutes. Remove from heat and stir in the basil. Serve topped with pecorino cheese.

NUTRITION

- 420 Calories
- 13g Total fat
- 12g Fiber
- 20g Protein

SNACK

MEDITERRANEAN CHICKPEA BOWL

PREPARATION TIME: 12 MIN   **COOKING TIME: 13 MIN**

SERVINGS: 2

INGREDIENTS

- ½ tbs. of cumin seeds
- 1 large julienned carrot
- A ¼ cup of tomatoes (chopped)
- 1 medium julienned zucchini
- A ¼ cup of lemon juice
- 2 sliced green chilies
- ¼ cup of olive oil
- A ½ cup of chopped parsley leaves
- 1 minced clove of garlic
- ¼ tbs. salt
- ¼ tbs. cayenne pepper powder
- A ¼ cup of radish (sliced)
- 3 tbs. walnuts (chopped)
- 1/3 feta cheese (crumbled)
- 1 big can of chickpeas
- Proportionate salad greens

DIRECTIONS

1. Another ingredient that you will see on the Mediterranean Diet list is chickpeas. The Mediterranean Chickpea Bowl is a popular snack that can be enjoyed at all times. You can use fresh or canned chickpeas as per preference.
2. For the salad, you will have to make a special dressing that will make the dish tasty. You need to roast the cumin seeds on a dry pan. Make sure the heat is at medium.
3. When the seeds begin releasing the aroma, put the seeds in a different mixing bowl. In this bowl, add the olive oil, garlic, lemon juice, and tomatoes. Also, add the cayenne pepper and salt, and mix well to blend in all the ingredients.
4. Take a big bowl and add the chickpeas into it. Then put in the sliced and chopped veggies, and parsley leaves.
5. Adding walnut pieces will add an extra crunch to the Mediterranean chickpea salad. Put in the seasoning you just prepared and then, mix all the ingredients well.

NUTRITION

- Carbohydrate – 30g
- Protein - 12g
- Fat – 38g
- Calories: 492

MEDITERRANEAN FLATBREAD WITH TOPPINGS

PREPARATION TIME: **10 MIN**   COOKING TIME: **15 MIN**

SERVINGS: **3**

INGREDIENTS

- 2 medium tomatoes
- 5 black olives (diced)
- 8 ounces of crescent rolls
- 1 clove of garlic (finely chopped)
- 1 red onion (sliced)
- ¼ tbs. salt
- 4 tbs. olive oil
- ¼ tbs. pepper powder
- 1 and ½ tbs. Italian seasoning
- Parmesan cheese as per requirement

DIRECTIONS

1. Wash and clean the tomatoes properly. Then make very thin and round slices with a sharp knife. You have to ensure that the tomato juices drain out. So, place these on a dry piece of linen cloth.
2. You will get crescent rolls or flatbread dough in the market. Unroll these and keep these on a big baking tray. Make sure the surface of the baking dish has no grease or water.
3. Then roll the dough into several portions, which will not be more than 14x10 inches in measurement.
4. With the help of a rolling pin, shape these into rectangular flatbreads.
5. Place the tomato slices, diced black olive and onion slices on these flatbreads.
6. Add the Italian seasoning, olive oil, pepper powder, salt, and chopped garlic together and mix well.
7. Take the mixture and apply an even coat on all the flatbreads. This mixture will add flavor to the toppings and flatbreads.
8. Put the baking tray in the microwave oven and set the temperature at 375°.
9. After 15 minutes, remove the plate from the oven and enjoy your crunchy Mediterranean flatbread with toppings with a glass of red wine.

NUTRITION

- Carbohydrate – 9g
- Protein - 2g
- Fat – 6g
- Calories: 101

CUCUMBER BITES

INGREDIENTS

- 1 English cucumber, sliced into 32 rounds
- 10 ounces hummus
- 16 cherry tomatoes, halved
- 1 tablespoon parsley, chopped
- 1 ounce feta cheese, crumbled

DIRECTIONS

1. Spread the hummus on each cucumber round, divide the tomato halves on each, sprinkle the cheese and parsley on to and serve as an appetizer.

NUTRITION

- Calories 162,
- Fat 3.4,
- Fiber 2,
- Carbs 6.4,
- Protein 2.4

STUFFED AVOCADO

PREPARATION TIME: 10 MIN   **COOKING TIME: 0 MIN**

SERVINGS: 2

INGREDIENTS

- 1 avocado, halved and pitted
- 10 ounces canned tuna, drained
- 2 tablespoons sun-dried tomatoes, chopped
- 1 and ½ tablespoon basil pesto
- 2 tablespoons black olives, pitted and chopped
- Salt and black pepper to the taste
- 2 teaspoons pine nuts, toasted and chopped
- 1 tablespoon basil, chopped

DIRECTIONS

1. In a bowl, combine the tuna with the sun-dried tomatoes and the rest of the ingredients except the avocado and stir.
2. Stuff the avocado halves with the tuna mix and serve as an appetizer.

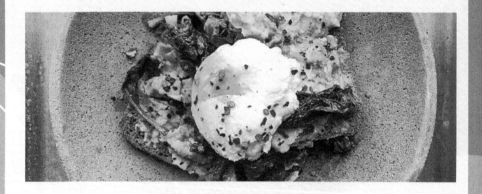

NUTRITION

- Calories 233,
- Fat 9,
- Fiber 3.5,
- Carbs 11.4,
- Protein 5.6

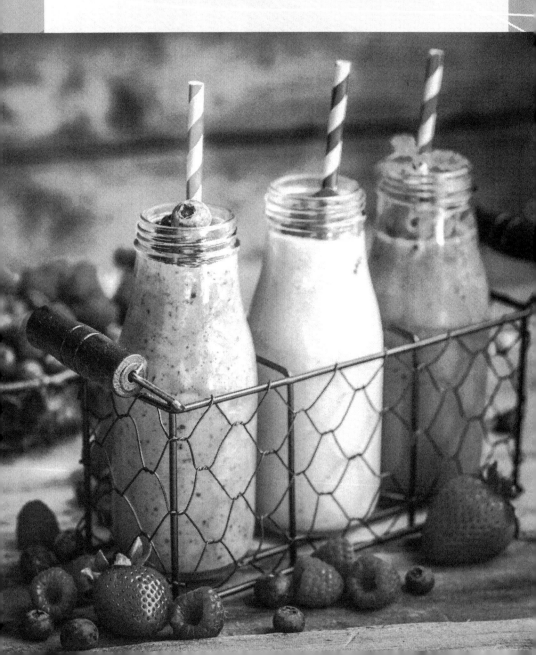

CHAPTER 10
SMOOTHIES AND DRINKS RECIPES

LUCKY MINT SMOOTHIE

PREPARATION TIME: 5 MIN　　　　　**COOKING TIME: 0 MIN**

SERVINGS: 2

INGREDIENTS

- 2 cups plant-based milk (here or here)
- 2 frozen bananas, halved
- 1 tbsp. fresh mint leaves or ¼ tsp. peppermint extract
- 1 tsp. vanilla extract

DIRECTIONS

1. In a blender, combine the milk, bananas, mint, and vanilla.
2. Blend on high for 1 to 2 minutes, or until the contents reach a smooth and creamy consistency, and serve.

VARIATION TIP: If you like to sneak greens into smoothies, add a cup or two of spinach to boost the health benefits of this smoothie and give it an even greener appearance.

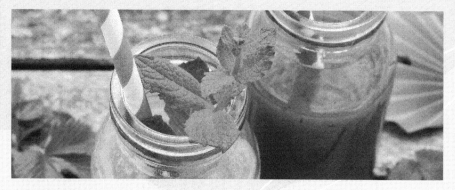

NUTRITION

- Calories: 182

PARADISE ISLAND SMOOTHIE

PREPARATION TIME: **5 MIN**   COOKING TIME: **0 MIN**

SERVINGS: **2**

INGREDIENTS

- 2 cups plant-based milk (here or here)
- 1 frozen banana
- ½ cup frozen mango chunks
- ½ cup frozen pineapple chunks
- 1 tsp. vanilla extract

DIRECTIONS

1. In a blender, combine the milk, banana, mango, pineapple, and vanilla.
2. Blend on high for 1 to 2 minutes, or until the contents reach a smooth and creamy consistency, and serve.

LEFTOVER TIP: If you have any leftover smoothies, you can put it in a jar with some rolled oats and allow the mixture to soak in the refrigerator overnight to create a tropical version of overnight oats.

NUTRITION

- Calories: 206

BUBBLY ORANGE SODA

PREPARATION TIME: **5 MIN**   COOKING TIME: **0 MIN**

SERVINGS: **2**

INGREDIENTS

- 4 cups carbonated water
- 2 cups pulp-free orange juice (4 oranges, freshly squeezed and strained)

DIRECTIONS

1. For each serving, pour 2 parts carbonated water and 1-part orange juice over ice right before serving.
2. Stir and enjoy it.

SERVING TIP: This recipe; is best made right before drinking. The amount of fizz in the carbonated water will decrease the longer it's open, so if you're going to make it ahead of time, make sure it's stored in an airtight, refrigerator-safe container.

NUTRITION

- Calories: 86

APPLE PIE SMOOTHIE

PREPARATION TIME: **5 MIN**   COOKING TIME: **0 MIN**

SERVINGS: **2**

INGREDIENTS

- 2 sweet crisp apples, cut into 1-inch cubes
- 2 cups plant-based milk (here or here)
- 1 cup ice
- 1 tbsp. maple syrup
- 1 tsp. ground cinnamon
- 1 tsp. vanilla extract

DIRECTIONS

1. In a blender, combine the apples, milk, ice, maple syrup, cinnamon, and vanilla
2. Blend on high for 1 to 2 minutes, or until the contents reach a smooth and creamy consistency, and serve.

VARIATION TIP: You can also use this recipe for making overnight oatmeal. Blend your smoothie, mix it with 2 cups rolled oats, and refrigerate overnight for a premade breakfast for two.

NUTRITION

- Calories: 228

VITAMIN GREEN SMOOTHIE

PREPARATION TIME: **5 MIN**   COOKING TIME: **5 MIN**

SERVINGS: **2**

INGREDIENTS

- 1 cup milk or juice
- 1 cup spinach or kale
- ½ cup plain yogurt
- 1 kiwi
- 1 tbsp. chia or flax
- 1 tsp. vanilla

DIRECTIONS

1. Mix the milk or juice and greens until smooth. Add the remaining ingredients and continue blending until smooth again.
2. Enjoy your delicious drink!

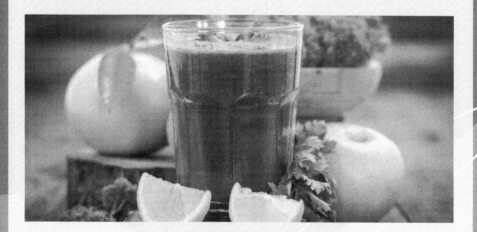

NUTRITION

- Calories: 397

STRAWBERRY GRAPEFRUIT SMOOTHIE

PREPARATION TIME: **5 MIN**   COOKING TIME: **5 MIN**

SERVINGS: **2**

INGREDIENTS

- 1 banana
- ½ cup strawberries, frozen
- 1 grapefruit
- ¼ cup milk
- ¼ cup plain yogurt
- 2 tbsp. honey
- ½ tsp. ginger, chopped

DIRECTIONS

1. Using a mixer, blend all the ingredients.
2. When smooth, top your drink with a slice of grapefruit and enjoy it!

NUTRITION

- Calories: 233

HOMEMADE OAT MILK

PREPARATION TIME: 5 MIN   **COOKING TIME: 0 MIN**

SERVINGS: 8

INGREDIENTS

- 1 cup rolled oats
- 4 cups of water

DIRECTIONS

1. Put the oats in a medium bowl, and cover with cold water. Soak for 15 minutes, then drain and rinse the oats.
2. Pour the cold water and the soaked oats into a blender. Blend for 60 to 90 seconds, or just until the mixture is creamy; white color throughout. (Blending any further; may over-blend the oats, resulting in gummy milk.)
3. Strain through a nut-milk bag or colander, then store in the refrigerator for up to 5 days.

VARIATION TIP: This recipe can easily be made into chocolate oat milk. Once you've strained the milk, return it to a blender with 3 tablespoons cocoa powder, 2 tablespoons maple syrup, and 1 teaspoon vanilla extract, then blend for 30 seconds.

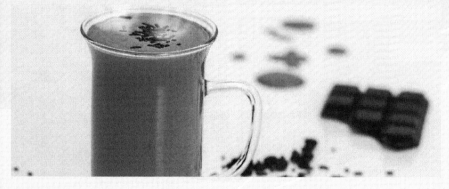

NUTRITION

- Calories: 69

CREAMY CASHEW MILK

PREPARATION TIME: **5 MIN**   COOKING TIME: **0 MIN**

SERVINGS: **8**

INGREDIENTS

- 4 cups of water
- ¼ cup raw cashews, soaked overnight

DIRECTIONS

1. In a blender, blend the water and cashews at high speed for 2 minutes.
2. Strain with a nut-milk bag or cheesecloth, then store in the refrigerator for up to 5 days.

VARIATION TIP: This recipe makes unsweetened cashew milk that can be used in savory and sweet dishes. For a creamier version to put in your coffee, cut the amount of water in half. For a sweeter version, add 1 to 2 tablespoons maple syrup and 1 teaspoon vanilla extract before blending.

NUTRITION

- Calories: 48

WATERMELON LEMONADE

PREPARATION TIME: 5 MIN   **COOKING TIME: 0 MIN**

SERVINGS: 6

INGREDIENTS

- 4 cups diced watermelon
- 4 cups cold water
- 2 tbsp. freshly squeezed lemon juice
- 1 tbsp. freshly squeezed lime juice

DIRECTIONS

1. In a blender, combine the watermelon, water, lemon juice, and lime juice, and blend for 1 minute.
2. Strain the contents through a fine-mesh sieve or nut-milk bag. Serve chilled. Store in the refrigerator; for up to 3 days.

SERVING TIP: Slice up a few lemons or lime wedges to serve with your Watermelon Lemonade, or top it with a few fresh mints leaves to give it an extra-crisp, minty flavor.

When it comes to refreshing summertime drinks, lemonade is always near the top of the list. This Watermelon "Lemonade" is perfect for using up leftover watermelon or for those early fall days when stores and farmers are almost giving them away. You can also substitute 4 cups of ice for the cold water to create a delicious summertime slushy.

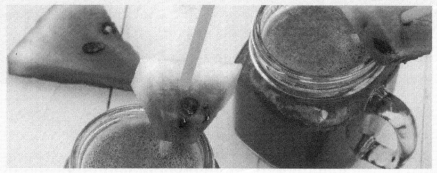

NUTRITION

- Calories: 90

CONCLUSION

If this has taught you anything, the hope is that it has taught you how many variables are involved when it comes to health and wellness. This aimed to share with you the plethora of options that are available to you when it comes to intermittent fasting and autophagy, as well as how to induce it within the cells of your body in order to achieve desired results and outcomes.

Think back on the many options that were laid out for you in this book involving diet options and specific foods that have the ability to induce autophagy in the brain. It is your job now to decide which of these foods or supplements to include in your life and to practice a sort of trial and error, noting which ones make you feel great and which ones you prefer to go without. With all of this information, you can decide which ways fit best with your specific lifestyle and your preferences.

As you can see, there are many different ways to optimize autophagy. The way or ways that you choose will be highly dependent on you as an individual. You may want to approach this by trying one and being open to changing methods if it does not work as well as you would like. You may want to try a combination of methods in order to get the best results. The key is to be flexible and be open to change, as nobody knows how their body will react to changes in diet and exercise.

In anything new that we try, there is a chance that we may fall off track. Fasting or following a new diet plan is no different. The focus should not be on the fact that you fell off but on how you decide to come back and approach it again. You need not give up altogether if you have a day or two where you did not accomplish your full fast. You just need to re-examine your plan and approach it in a different way. Maybe your fasting period was too long for your first try. Maybe your fasting and eating windows did not match up with your sleep-wake cycle as well as they could have. Any of these factors can be adjusted to suit your lifestyle needs better and make fasting or a specific diet work for you. With the human body, there is never a right or a wrong way to approach anything; there is only a multitude of different ways, and some that will be better for your specific body and mind than others. Being open to trying different variations and adjusting your plan as you go can be the difference between success and decided to give up.

If you fall off track, scale your plan back a little bit and try it again. If you are worried that you are not doing enough, begin with the scaled-back plan and get used to this first. You can always increase your fasting times later on once you know you are completely comfortable with a shorter fasting time.

As you can see, there are numerous benefits that come with employing an intermittent fasting diet. I promised you that within these pages you would find out why your body reacts differently to diet programs and how you can deal with it, and that I would provide you with specific examples of intermittent fasting programs that were designed with your sex and age in mind. After reading this, you now have this information and much, much more! You are fully equipped to begin changing your life with programs designed specifically for you, and I hope that you feel empowered to do so!

The main takeaway is that there are many options for women over the age of 50 to take control of their weight loss strategies, without having to turn to methods designed for men or people in their twenties. Further, taking control of your health and playing an active role in your disease risk reduction is not as difficult as it sounds. I hope that after reading this, you have a new understanding of what you can do and how your body will react given your age and sex.

As you take all of this information forth with you, it may seem overwhelming to begin applying this to your own life. Remember, life is a process, and you do not need to expect perfection from yourself. By reading this, you are already on your way to changing your life.

SOURCES

Life in the fasting lane, Jason Fung, Eve Mayer, Megan Ramos, HarperCollins Books 2019

The switch, James W. Clement, Gallery Books 2019

The longevity diet, Valter Longo, Avery 2018

The science and fine arts of fasting, Herbert M. Shelton, Martino Fine Books 2013

Natural Hygiene: Man's pristine way of life, Herbert M. Shelton, Dodo Press 2005

Fasting can save your Life, Herbert M. Shelton, and Ronald G. Cridland, American Natural Hygiene Society, 1978

21 DAYS MEAL PLAN & INTERACTIVE PLANNER

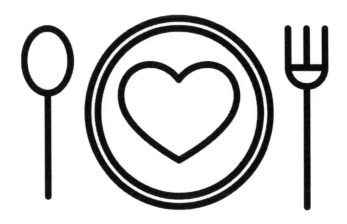

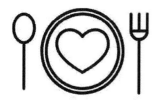

MEAL PLAN
GENERAL RULES

21 day plan is to be implemented gradually, because the body needs time to adjust to the lower amount of food

A meal plan ensures a correct distribution of carbs, proteins, fats and vitamins

When possible, it is best to use fresh and seasonal vegetables and fruit

Anytime you are too busy or too tired to cook you can choose a serving of fresh fruit or a fruit smoothie

Try to choose best quality and organic food when possible, opting for fresh foods instead of processed ones

Try to avoid carbs (like pasta, pizza and bread) for dinner, reducing sugar consumption before bedtime

Include some fruits and vegetables every day

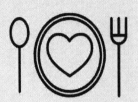

WEEK 1
MEAL PLAN
SPONTANEOUS OMISSION METHOD

S
- BREAKFAST: sausage omelet — 334 kal
- LUNCH: easy mayo salmon — 133 kal
- SNACK: mediterranean flat bread with toppings — 267 kal
- DINNER: apple pie smoothie — 228 kal

M
- BREAKFAST: buckwheat buttermilk pancakes — 108 kal
- LUNCH: pasta puttanesca — 383 kal
- SNACK: keto coconut flake balls — 204 kal
- **DINNER: FAST**

T
- BREAKFAST: quinoa fruit salad — 159 kal
- LUNCH: mediterranean instant pot shredded beef — 190.2 kal
- SNACK: cucumber bites — 162 kal
- DINNER: grilled veggie skewers — 680 kal

W
- BREAKFAST: delicious turkey wrap — 162 kal
- LUNCH: zesty avocado and lettuce salad — 125.7 kal
- SNACK: vitamin green smoothie — 397 kal
- DINNER: butternut squash risotto — 140 kal

TH
- BREAKFAST: mixed berries oatmeal with sweet vanilla cream — 150 kal
- LUNCH: shrimps with lemon and pepper + roasted vegetables — 185 kal
- SNACK: borek with spinach filling — 219 kal
- **DINNER: FAST**

F
- BREAKFAST: mediterranean pita breakfast — 267 kal
- LUNCH: thai green curry with spring vegatebles — 140 kal
- SNACK: creamy cashew milk — 48 kal
- DINNER: tuna and potato salad — 406 kal

S
- BREAKFAST: chickpea omelet with spinach and mushrooms — 147 kal
- LUNCH: pasta with pesto — 405 kal
- SNACK: stuffed avocado — 233 kal
- **DINNER: FAST**

**Calories in this plan are only a guide to ensure you do not exceed 1000 kcal per day
This is necessary to prepare the body for fasting**

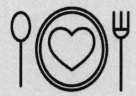

WEEK 2
MEAL PLAN
5 : 2 PROTOCOL

S
- BREAKFAST: pumpkin pancakes — *500 kal day* — 70 kal
- LUNCH: broccoli and turkey dish — 120 kal
- SNACK: lucky mint smoothie — 182 kal
- DINNER: brown rice stir fry with vegetables — 140 kal

M
- BREAKFAST: mediterranean pita breakfast
- LUNCH: pasta with creamy tomato sauce
- SNACK: chipotle and lime tortilla chips
- DINNER: cilantro lime flounder

T
- BREAKFAST: quinoa black bean breakfast bowl
- LUNCH: keto buffalo chicken empanadas
- SNACK: creamy spinach
- DINNER: traditional chicken vegetable soup

W
- BREAKFAST: French toast with almonds and peach compote
- LUNCH: eggplant fettuccine or spaghetti pasta
- SNACK: avocado fries
- DINNER: tuna and potato salad

TH
- BREAKFAST: vegan muffins breakfast sandwich — *500 kal day* — 235 kal
- LUNCH: honey roasted cauliflower — 88 kal
- SNACK: creamy cashew milk — 58 kal
- DINNER: thai green curry with spring vegetables — 140 kal

F
- BREAKFAST: almond waffles with cranberries
- LUNCH: shrimps with lemon and pepper
- SNACK: zucchini hummus
- DINNER: eggplant teryiaki bowl

S
- BREAKFAST: corn griddlecakes with tofu mayonnaise
- LUNCH: pepperoni and cheddar Stromboli
- SNACK: creamy spinach
- DINNER: herb pesto tuna

In this plan, calories are important only for the two days that you do not exceed 500 kal

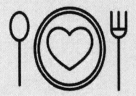

WEEK 3
MEAL PLAN
16: 8 METHOD

S
- BREAKFAST: **FAST**
- LUNCH: basil coconut peas and broccoli
- SNACK: carrot and sweet potato fritters
- DINNER: quinoa and black beans chili

M
- BREAKFAST: **FAST**
- LUNCH: cheesy caprese salad
- SNACK: polenta skewers
- DINNER: baked orzo with eggplant, swiss chard and mozzarella

T
- BREAKFAST: **FAST**
- LUNCH: chickpea with spinach and mushrooms
- SNACK: bell pepper nachos
- DINNER: barley risotto with tomatoes

W
- BREAKFAST: **FAST**
- LUNCH: pasta puttanesca
- SNACK: borek with spinach filling
- DINNER: grilled calamari with lemon and herbs

TH
- BREAKFAST: **FAST**
- LUNCH: mediterranean instant pot shredded beef
- SNACK: cucumber bites
- DINNER: chickpeas and kale with spicy pomodoro sauce

F
- BREAKFAST: **FAST**
- LUNCH: pasta puttanesca
- SNACK: stuffed avocado
- DINNER: cilantro lime flounder

S
- BREAKFAST: **FAST**
- LUNCH: zesty avocado and lettuce salad
- SNACK: mediterranean flatbread with with toppings
- DINNER: sweet potatoes

In this plan it is not necessary to count calories since you are respecting 16 hours fasting every day. Just be sure to chose healthy and well balanced food.

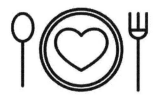

INTERACTIVE
MEAL PLAN

INSTRUCTIONS

In the first section of your weekly calendar:

- Write the name of the fasting methods you decide to follow during the week
- Put an X on the days and meals you plan to fast.

In the second section specify:

- Your goal for the week
- The results obtained at the end of the week
- The lbs lost during the week
- Notes on what aspects can be improved

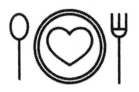

STARTING POINT

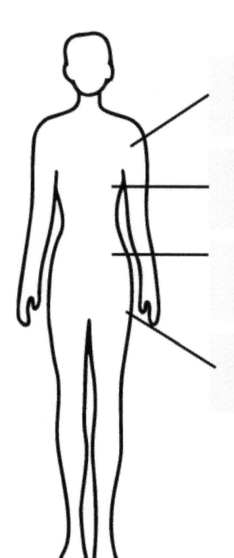

ARMS
inches
....

CHEST
inches
....

WAIST
inches
....

HIPS
inches
....

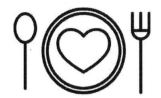

WEEKLY FASTING PLAN

WEEK 1			
FASTING METHOD			
	BREAKFAST	**LUNCH**	**DINNER**
Monday			
Tuesday			
Wednesday			
Thursday			
Friday			
Saturday			
Sunday			

GOAL	
ACCOMPLISHMENT	
LBS LOST	
TO BE IMPROVED	

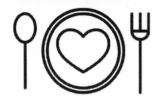

WEEKLY
FASTING PLAN

WEEK 2			
FASTING METHOD			
	BREAKFAST	**LUNCH**	**DINNER**
Monday			
Tuesday			
Wednesday			
Thursday			
Friday			
Saturday			
Sunday			

GOAL	
ACCOMPLISHMENT	
LBS LOST	
TO BE IMPROVED	

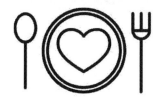

WEEKLY FASTING PLAN

WEEK 3			
FASTING METHOD			
	BREAKFAST	**LUNCH**	**DINNER**
Monday			
Tuesday			
Wednesday			
Thursday			
Friday			
Saturday			
Sunday			

GOAL	
ACCOMPLISHMENT	
LBS LOST	
TO BE IMPROVED	

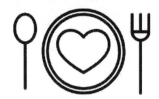

WEEKLY FASTING PLAN

WEEK 4			
FASTING METHOD			
	BREAKFAST	**LUNCH**	**DINNER**
Monday			
Tuesday			
Wednesday			
Thursday			
Friday			
Saturday			
Sunday			

GOAL	
ACCOMPLISHMENT	
LBS LOST	
TO BE IMPROVED	

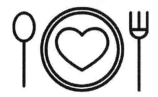

WEEKLY FASTING PLAN

WEEK 5			
FASTING METHOD			
	BREAKFAST	**LUNCH**	**DINNER**
Monday			
Tuesday			
Wednesday			
Thursday			
Friday			
Saturday			
Sunday			

GOAL	
ACCOMPLISHMENT	
LBS LOST	
TO BE IMPROVED	

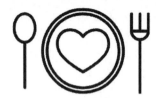

WEEKLY FASTING PLAN

WEEK 6			
FASTING METHOD			
	BREAKFAST	**LUNCH**	**DINNER**
Monday			
Tuesday			
Wednesday			
Thursday			
Friday			
Saturday			
Sunday			

GOAL	
ACCOMPLISHMENT	
LBS LOST	
TO BE IMPROVED	